RARE

A Journey of Self-Acceptance

by

Zoë Bull

**Grosvenor House
Publishing Limited**

This book is published by
Grosvenor House Publishing Ltd
Link House
140 The Broadway, Tolworth, Surrey, KT6 7HT.
www.grosvenorhousepublishing.co.uk

A CIP record for this book
is available from the British Library

ISBN 978-1-83975-523-1

*"The flower that blooms in adversity is
the most rare and beautiful of all"*
(The Emperor, Mulan)

CONTENTS

FOREWORD

I had the pleasure of meeting Zoë in my Tuberous Sclerosis clinic many moons ago. I recall her positivity and determination not to be defined or limited by the condition which affected so many aspects of her life.

My name is Dr Sam Amin, I am a consultant paediatric neurologist with a special interest in Tuberous Sclerosis Complex (TSC). I have been treating adults and children with TSC for many years. TSC is fascinating and unique in that it is one of the few genetic conditions that we have learnt a lot about within the early years of this new genetic era. We have identified an exact molecular defect, which has helped us to develop targeted therapies.

There is a significant, supportive TSC community made up of sufferers and their families, whom, alongside health professionals working in the field, have worked tirelessly to improve the lives and opportunities for TSC sufferers.

The natural history of TSC is already changing. Sadly, in the past, many people lost their lives from TSC related complications. If the complications were not fatal, they often still resulted in significant morbidity, including the loss of function of body organs, or severe long-term learning disabilities. I am confident and hopeful that in the next decade it will be rare to see these complications in individuals with TSC. TSC is becoming a disease which is easier to modify. It is exciting to be part of this positive change.

Zoë had a very difficult journey with her TSC related complications. I cannot stress enough how important Zoë's coping mechanisms have been in surmounting all the hurdles she has been faced with. Her book highlights these challenges and how she managed to overcome them. The book is a good description of many of the most amazing people I have encountered through my career who live with TSC. And while they may have different difficulties in life, they all share a similar path. This book captures the reality of a life touched by TSC and will be an encouragement to those who read it. Zoë has achieved so much, in spite of all that was stacked against her.

Despite all her battles, Zoë agreed to take part in an experimental drug trial. Zoë was aware that there was a 50% chance that she may be given a placebo, but she was prepared to go through with extra tests and assessments because she understood that her contribution had the potential to further change the lives of many individuals with TSC.

I have read and written several scientific papers and book chapters on TSC in my professional capacity, however, Zoë's book has given me a deeper insight into TSC, from a different angle. I feel very privileged to be part of her journey.

Dr Sam Amin

REFLECTIONS – A SUMMARY OF ACCEPTANCE

This book has been about developing self-acceptance. It hasn't always been easy to write, but I knew that I wanted to. In December 2014, I was in the midst of a dark period of ill-health in hospital. I knew that if I wrote a book about TS and LAM, then people with the conditions would feel less alone, that self-acceptance is possible despite the odds, and that I could help raise awareness to the general population about these very rare health conditions.

Self-acceptance is something that we all strive for, and therefore connects us all. I remember reaching that point of self-acceptance, like I had reached the top of a mountain, yet thinking, do I just walk down from here?

But after some reflection, I began viewing this level of self-acceptance as a new baseline to exist from, as part of a life-long process. I can recognise my imperfections, yet still feel content. I can acknowledge TS and LAM are parts of me, but I have a strong sense of normality as well. I'm a fluid, yet whole person.

Zoë
July, 2020

ACKNOWLEDGEMENTS

Thank you to all the people who have supported me or taken an interest in developing research for these two very rare diseases: Tuberous Sclerosis Complex and LAM.

Thank you, Dr Keast, for knowing what TSC was in the 1990s and being able to diagnose me, as well as being a caring and amusing GP for me and my family.

Thank you to the staff at the TSC Clinic at the Royal United Hospital in Bath, including: Professor Osborne and Professor O'Callaghan, as well as Dr Amin, who supported me through the medical trial I took part in, and kindly wrote the foreword for Rare.

Thank you to Professor Johnson for dedicating so much of your career into the research of LAM, as well as having such a kind medical team at the National LAM Centre in Nottingham.

Thank you to the additional hospitals who have looked after me either as a patient or an outpatient: the paediatric team at the Royal Berkshire Hospital, noting Dr Newman; the neurology department at the John Radcliffe Hospital, involving Dr Lennox; thoracic surgeons, Mr Routledge and Mr Pilling and their teams on the thoracic ward at Guy's Hospital, and the medical professionals who were involved in my emergency embolisation surgery at the Royal Berks.

To the Tuberous Sclerosis Association (TSA) for all your research into the condition and creating a supportive community for all kinds of TSC-affected people. Thank you to the CEO, Louise Fish, for reading through my book before it was published.

Thank you to LAM Action for giving me the opportunity to meet other people with the condition and to Jill Pateman, Gill Hollis and Professor Anne Tattersfield for proofreading the details on LAM.

To Mencap, who have given me my first job and helped me to understand people affected by learning disabilities. Thank you to my manager and friend, Maddella, for always looking out for me and supporting me unconditionally.

Thank you to all my honorary family members, The Daveys, and Vivien being a trusted advisor during my counselling training. Thank you, Eric and Betty, for nursing me back to health when I had bronchitis and for the wonderful long chats over a nice cup of tea.

To all my friends I have grown up with and who have accepted my conditions, and have stood by me when I have been unwell, and to those who have allowed me to write about them in this book.

Thank you to Talking Therapies for providing beneficial Cognitive Behavioural Therapy and to Catherine who really helped me to look TSC and LAM in the eye, during my counselling training.

Thank you, Grosvenor House Publishing, for giving me the opportunity to self-publish my work and share my story.

Finally, a big thank you to Mum, Dad, Geoffrey and Sarah. I am so grateful that you are my family and for the unconditional love that you give me; allowing me to thrive, supporting me at my appointments, and helping me achieve my dreams.

INTRODUCTION

Anomaly

I'm an anomaly. Look up in the dictionary what an anomaly is, and that pretty much describes me.

"Something that deviates from what is standard, normal or expected"

From the word go, when I was being created, somewhere I must have decided that I wanted to do things differently. Why just be normal, when I could have a rare condition called Tuberous Sclerosis Complex (TSC), that no one else in my family has ever had, and whilst I'm at it, I could challenge all the common misconceptions about people who have some form of disability along the way.

I can only imagine it was like a pick 'n' mix kind of event with the irony that I couldn't consciously choose what I wanted. I went to a TSC charity event one year in my early twenties and a group of us took part in a workshop that involved picking up an object that represented our personal journeys. I reached out to pick a pink swirly shell, but another person grabbed it. Having to accept the matter, I chose another shell, but I wouldn't have picked it up otherwise.

If I consciously had the decision to have TSC, I probably wouldn't have taken it. I would have chosen that seemingly perfect shell over the other normal looking one with its slight imperfections. But seeing that the shell now sits on my bookcase, I'm grateful that I do have some unique experiences that I will be sharing throughout this book.

When I think back to those common misconceptions I was talking about, I'm guilty to admit that I have misjudged other people with health conditions too. There have been times that I thought everyone with TSC had a learning disability apart from me, and that if I didn't know what it was like to experience epilepsy, then I would assume any epileptic person would be rolling around on the floor uncontrollably, but actually that is not always the case – they might feel a bit nauseous and lightheaded for a few moments, before continuing life as normal.

People with any kind of health condition have feelings, emotions and desires that any other person in the world has. We all deserve that. So, if I mention some of my judgments throughout this book, then I can only apologise if feelings are hurt, but that is not intentional or personal towards anyone. My words are simply recollections of times that have challenged me coming to terms with having two connected health conditions myself.

Throughout this book are both chapters on science and personal experience. They can be read as individual sections or a chronological story of my development. As the official title of the primary disease is called Tuberous Sclerosis Complex, I have mentioned it as TSC in the factual sections of the book. However, as I have grown up calling it Tuberous Sclerosis, I have referred to it as TS in my personal reflections.

But what is it?

What is Tuberous Sclerosis Complex

One million people worldwide are born with a rare genetic condition called Tuberous Sclerosis Complex (TSC). That is on average every 1 in 6,000 births.

The *sclerosis* part of the condition may sound familiar, such as in Multiple Sclerosis (MS). As an overall term, sclerosis refers to the *overgrowth of fibrous tissue,* which can harden. In MS the hardened tissue, known as plaques, can form scars on the brain or spinal cord that damage the function of nerves in the central nervous system. However, in Tuberous Sclerosis Complex the nature of the condition leans more towards the overgrowth of the non-cancerous fibrous tissue on various organs: the brain, skin, heart, eyes, kidneys and lungs. It's important to note though, that Multiple Sclerosis and Tuberous Sclerosis Complex are not connected diseases.

How a person can be affected by TSC is connected to which organs may have these growths, generally known as *tubers.* Some people may have tubers in all the organs listed above whereas other people may have one or two organs that are affected. The size of the tubers can also influence the severity of how a person is affected by TSC. One person might have severe epilepsy and learning disabilities, whereas another may have an overgrowth of skin cells on their face and an average IQ. The condition varies from person to person.

Genes

As a genetic disorder, Tuberous Sclerosis Complex occurs at conception rather than as a contagious disease that could be passed between people. The UK's leading charity in TSC is the Tuberous Sclerosis Association (TSA) who describe our genes as being part of our DNA – an instruction manual for how our bodies work, with details we may or may not have inherited from our parents.

However, with genetic disorders, unexpected changes can happen when the *instruction manual* is being created and can cause diseases like TSC. The genes involved with Tuberous Sclerosis Complex include TSC1 and TSC2 that contain proteins called hamartin (TSC1) and tuberin (TSC2). Both of these proteins influence the development of cells, including the size of the cells and how fast they grow. For people who are not affected by Tuberous Sclerosis Complex, the hamartin and tuberin work in harmony, collaboratively monitoring the development of cells so they grow at a gradual and controlled rate. If there is an error in either the TSC1 or TSC2 genes, then this can cause cells to divide or grow uncontrollably, which causes the benign tumours and Tuberous Sclerosis Complex to develop.

Inherited or Sporadic?

Despite Tuberous Sclerosis Complex being a genetic condition, only a third of people affected have inherited it from either or both parents. In these cases, it is often the TSC1 gene that has been altered, whereas unexpected changes in the TSC2 can cause a randomised version of TSC known as sporadic Tuberous Sclerosis Complex. This spontaneous version means that neither parent or previous relative has carried faulty TSC genes and the child will be the first in their bloodline to have the disease.

In very rare cases, 3 percent of parents unaffected by the condition, can carry the faulty genes in their sperm or eggs, but nowhere else in the body. This can mean one child could be born without developing TSC, whereas the following child may have had the faulty genes passed onto them. This is known as germline mosaicism.

Connections to LAM

Faults in the TSC1 and TSC2 genes can also play a part in development of a sister disease known as Lymphangioleimyomatosis (LAM) which affects 30% of people with Tuberous Sclerosis Complex. The large majority of cases are believed to be women, with medical research suggesting that the hormone oestrogen can influence the development of the disease.

As with TSC, women with LAM have problematic cell growth which is localised to the respiratory system, kidneys and lymphatic system. This means that cysts develop in the lungs, potentially causing breathing issues, lung collapses, or bleeding in the kidneys.

Other similarities that this lung disease shares with Tuberous Sclerosis Complex, is that LAM can also occur sporadically, as a stand-alone condition. Depending on the DNA recipe of each person, one woman might have a mixture of healthy and faulty TSC1 and TSC2 genes, which means she could just develop sporadic LAM, or just have Tuberous Sclerosis Complex. In other cases, some women develop both conditions known as TSC-related LAM.

A detailed chapter on Lymphangioleimyomatosis (LAM) is featured later in the book.

CHAPTER 1

THE BRAIN: TSC & EPILEPSY

Approximately 80% of people with TSC are affected by epilepsy. It is one of the first symptoms that shows often in infancy but can be diagnosed in childhood and adult life as well.

What is epilepsy?

Epilepsy Action describes it as being "one of the most common neurological conditions in the world" with the World Health Organisation (WHO) suggesting 50 million people of the general population are affected worldwide. About 600,000 of those people live in the UK.

Epilepsy shows itself in the form of seizures of which there are over forty different types.

"Electrical activity is happening in our brain all the time, as the cells in the brain send messages to each other. A seizure happens when there is a sudden burst of intense electrical activity in the brain. This causes a temporary disruption to the way the brain normally works, so the brain's messages become mixed up. The result is an epileptic seizure."

(Epilepsy Action)

The type of seizure depends on where in the brain the electrical disruption takes place. Activity can be localised to one area of the brain, which is called Focal-Aware Seizure. This type is the most common occurrence of epilepsy in TSC and involves a person remaining conscious of their surroundings but may feel a wave sensation come over them accompanied with light-headedness and a strange sense of smell or taste. Focal-Aware seizures last a few seconds to several minutes. These seizures on their own are sometimes referred to as Auras. Other times an Aura can spread to more generalised parts of the brain. This may include Focal Impaired Awareness seizures, where consciousness is affected. Tonic-clonic, Absences and Myclonic Seizures may also affect consciousness or cause the body to move involuntarily or go tense.

Causes of epilepsy and connections to TSC

Many people with seizures don't know what causes their epilepsy, but often there are links to genetics, brain damage or brain tumours. Epilepsy is common in Tuberous Sclerosis Complex because disorganised areas of the brain called Cortical Tubers can interrupt those electrical messages causing seizures.

Other abnormalities in a TSC-affected brain may include Subependymal nodules (SENs) that are fluid-filled cells around the brain that may need removal with surgery if they grow too big. Similarly, Subependymal Giant Cell Astrocytoma (SEGA) are non-cancerous brain tumours that may not cause any issues for people with TSC, but could influence brain development, causing learning disabilities, such as Autism. Depending on the individual, a person could have neither of these abnormalities but still have TSC. It could also be said that someone may have SENs but not a SEGA and vice-versa. Everyone with TSC is affected differently.

How is the brain monitored?

Cortical Tubers, SENs and SEGAs are monitored via an MRI (Magnetic Resonance Imaging) scan. The patient lies on a board that slides into the MRI machine, which involves radio waves and a magnetic field that the patient would not be able to feel. These forces create a visual image on a computer screen of the area being scanned. Depending on the organ or situation, the duration of the scan can take between fifteen minutes to over an hour.

My Experience

Diagnosis

1994

"Zoë's acting a bit strange," my nine-year-old sister, Sarah, observed to my parents who were in the front seats of the car. We were on holiday in Somerset and Geoffrey, my eleven-year-old brother, had also noticed that every so often my one-year-old body would tense up in my car seat between him and Sarah, and I would stare blankly into space.

Similar situations happened on the way home from my childminder. Mum took me to see our GP, Dr Keast, who informed her that I may have a rare condition called Tuberous Sclerosis Complex, and symptoms of epilepsy and white patches on my skin were key elements of the disease.

Although I don't remember being diagnosed, I do remember the paediatric appointments at the local hospital; a bright light shining in my eye, a small hammer bashing my knees and elbows testing out my reflexes, and my weight and height being monitored. I was also referred to the Royal United Hospital in Bath for specialist TSC treatment.

I hated missing a day off school to go to Bath and I always felt grumpy. The same medical observations taking place including blood pressure checks and MRI scans to monitor the size of the benign tumour in my brain. I was unaware though, why I was having to attend these appointments. I remember preparing for my first MRI scan with a colouring book about how the process works; *No way was I going to colour that in!*

Mum and Dad encouraged me to practice lying still on a rug in our lounge for half an hour with my favourite toy dog, Lisa. I did it, but it took a lot of effort for an eight-year-old not to wriggle. The scanner was noisy, like a mixture of cymbals bashing together and bursts of air being pumped through a tube in my ears. Not to mention it was claustrophobic. At least I could listen to my Avril Lavigne CD through a set of headphones, but even my music couldn't override the noise pollution.

<u>2003</u>

It was beautifully warm April evening in Florida. My parents and I were sitting one end of Mainstreet U.S.A at Tony's Lady and the Tramp Restaurant, staring at the sunset toned Cinderella castle in the distance. It was a wonderful time to be enjoying delicious spaghetti, and wine for my parents. I was enjoying the last week of being nine.

While I ate my meal and appreciated the view, a subtle warm fuzzy feeling came over me and I felt light-headed, the blood rushing to my legs. *Was I fainting or dying? What was this?*

I didn't share how I felt with my parents, I suppose I didn't want to scare them, but over the next two years, I began to have more and more of these funny feelings, without really knowing what they were and what was causing them. It filled me with panic.

4

I would sit in school, listening to my teacher and that familiar fuzzy feeling would come over me and I would lower my head, pretending to reach something from my school bag, while I encouraged the blood to flow back to my brain. This scary sensation would last about 30 seconds, before dissolving away and I would resume the rest of my day.

Most of the time, I remembered these sensations and felt a bit sick in my stomach and my heart rate would go up as part of the adrenaline rush; other times I wouldn't remember a thing. I would read out loud to Mum before bed and if I had a seizure, Mum would tell me that I stopped reading and gone quiet. I felt embarrassed and self-conscious.

2004

Some days I would have seizures, sometimes I wouldn't, but once I had an absence seizure in front of my childhood friend, Izzy. I was now eleven and we'd stopped playing with toys and turned to chatting as our main form of entertainment. One Friday evening when Izzy was around, I remember sitting on the stairs blurting out a question about what we were having for dinner. Mum and Dad were in front of me trying to calm me down.

After Izzy had gone home, my parents explained to me that I wasn't fully conscious for about half an hour. My brow furrowed in confusion, tears burning the backs of my eyes.

"You weren't able to talk, Zoë," says Mum concerned. "You were just looking at us, like a frightened animal unable to say anything, but your eyes looked so scared."

My parents contacted the hospital in Bath for some advice and arranged an appointment. I was learning that the strange sensations were seizures. I had epilepsy.

I was prescribed Carbamazepine, a common anti-epileptic drug, but I was still having seizures. In October we went to Boston for a family half-term holiday. The North American landscape in autumn was beautiful; the sparkling water in Walden Pond and the rich copper leaves on the grand trees were picturesque, but those holiday memories had been tainted with regular seizure activity.

After the holiday we went back to Bath and discovered with Professor Osborne that I was consuming a tropical juice drink at breakfast. Pineapple and grapefruit breakdown the enzymes in the medicine, influencing the positive impact of reducing my seizures. I also learnt that alcohol has milder but similar effect, so I reduced the amount of wine in my glass on a Sunday.

2008

By putting these new habits into practice, my epilepsy activity decreased dramatically, and I went for four years without having a seizure. In the August Izzy came on holiday to France with us and over that fortnight I was gradually reducing my Carbamazepine intake. Izzy had witnessed the worse seizure of my life and was now seeing me come off my medication. We celebrated with our favourite blackcurrant liqueur; Cassis mixed with lemonade.

2010

It was a relief to be seizure free for a few years and when I was seventeen, I was able to learn how to drive. I had been warned all those years ago that if I have seizure once I pass my test, then I may have to temporarily surrender my driving licence until I'm seizure free for one whole year.

I enjoyed learning to drive. Mum taught me in her Citroën car at home and I loved the feeling of changing gear and pressing my feet down on the pedals. It was great to have my hands on the wheel and control of the car.

2012

In June I passed my driving test on my second attempt. It was a wonderful feeling to have a licence, even if I didn't have my own car yet. Six months later, just before Christmas I had an appointment in Bath because my seizures had started again, and we discussed going back on medication.

2013

Within the first week of January, I got a letter from the DVLA to say that they had received my surrendered licence. I was too upset about it to write in my journal. Although I didn't write about it; I was filled with disappointment. I hated that my epilepsy had returned and had to acknowledge that it wouldn't be safe for me to drive. I couldn't risk that.

For the next few years I began a seizure journal to track any patterns. I tended to have some kind of a seizure every two weeks or in stressful times, and in holiday periods when I would allow my mind to relax.

2017

At the start of the year I began an additional prescription of medication, Rapamycin, also known as Sirolimus. The medicine helps to slow down the deterioration of the lungs but has benefits in reducing other tumours associated with TS, including in my brain. However, Rapamycin and Carbamazepine were beginning to fight against each other and give me some funny side effects.

2018

4th April 2018

It's 2am on our cruise and I just had a strange seizure. I had gone to the toilet, and as I opened the door the familiar sensation came over me, but when I came out of the seizure,

I was half-way down the main corridor, confused that I had left the room.

It makes sense though because I did something similar a few weeks ago in March. Again, I was going to the toilet, but then when I came around, I had walked downstairs and was sitting at the kitchen table with the light on, eating my breakfast. The clock read 1.45 am. I was just about to make my sandwiches...Have I been sleepwalking? How did I not fall down the stairs?

Within the next six months I continued to have similar sleepwalking experiences and was referred to a local Neurologist, Dr Lennox. He considered that I had perhaps had an initial seizure but that afterwards, as a result of my medication interacting, my body resumed in a semi-conscious state in that part of my brain was awake and part of it was still asleep. In October I began to take an alternative anti-epileptic medicine called Levetiracetam, that was known to have minimal side effects with other medications.

Initially, I felt drowsy, adjusting to my new medicine but between November 2018 to July 2019, I was seizure free and it was fantastic. I was four months away from being able to drive again after seven years.

22nd July 2019

When I woke up, I read a book in bed before crunching away at my cereal. After breakfast I turned on my laptop and began checking my emails. Around 8 am, I could feel an overstimulating sensation of negative energy which smoothly transitioned into a focal seizure. The feeling washed over me, my heart rate increased, and I felt a bit nauseous. I am very disappointed that I've let myself down. I cried. Mum hugged me.

16th August 2019

I'm cross I had another partial seizure this morning. It was only a small one, but it definitely was one. I began increasing my Levetiracetam up to 1000mg on Tuesday, but I suppose I have done quite well not having a seizure for almost a week.

Still, it's disappointing though and I feel I have let myself down again. I guess it is feeling out of control as I can't predict when seizures will happen; I could have one at any time. Worrying about having one seems to make more occur.

12th September 2019

I had two partial seizures today and sent a letter to my neurologist to see if he could see me again; it was back in March when he discharged me. I'm trying to accept my epilepsy. It's hard to not try and push it away, but acceptance is so powerful. Perhaps the main thing is to become less afraid of my epilepsy and then I won't be so anxious about seizures happening and that may reduce them? It's hard not to be afraid though.

5th December 2019

I know that medically my epilepsy is caused by TS and the SEGA in my brain. Epilepsy has affected me in different ways growing up but has been most active in times of stress. Sometimes I have seizures out of the blue but most often it has been when my cortisol levels have dropped in my pre-frontal cortex of my brain during holiday periods.

As far as I know, I have had seizures during times of change – external events such as transitioning from primary to secondary school, or internal changes such as hormones fluctuating in adolescence to adulthood.

It was a relief to discover that my SEGA had decreased in size since I had been on both Rapamycin and Levetiracetam. The results gave me reassurance that I'm in a stable condition which therefore decreased my seizures activity. Then when my next seizure came, I was filled with disappointment, realising I would have to wait yet another year before I could drive again.

I tried not to think about having seizures. I spoke to my counsellor who suggested that acknowledging that I have epilepsy, may help me to accept it. I considered that perhaps I had been too impatient about trying to get to that 365-day seizure free goal post, which was causing more stress and more seizures.

At the time I had a phone app where I could track my epilepsy activity. I realised that every time I unlocked my phone, I would be reminded of the previous seizure. I decided it was important to take a step back and just track my epilepsy on the app's website.

March 2020

As I tracked my seizures on the website over the past three months, I spotted that I would have an initial seizure around the middle of month and then become afraid of having more seizures. For the third week of each month there were notably more seizures as I tried to will myself not to have any. Towards the end of the week, my perceived seizure threat dissolved until I had the next unexpected seizure. Or was I predicting I would have another one around the middle of the following month?

I wondered whether the visual calendar image from the website was adding to my sense of control to avoid seizure activity. When I wrote my seizures in a notebook I wasn't as concerned about when my previous seizure was. Having the calendar image in my mind was perhaps causing my anxiety rather than reducing it?

I remembered from my Cognitive Behavioural Therapy (CBT) in 2013, that it was my resistance to anxiety that caused me to have more anxious feelings rather than less. When I allowed the anxiety to be present and not label it as a problem, it lost its fear factor in me.

26th March 2020

Today I read through my CBT folder and all the health anxiety modules I had covered. As epilepsy is health-related I wondered whether working through the modules again and inserting 'epilepsy' as my main fear would help me challenge my negative associations with it. I decided to make an epilepsy CBT folder.

I identified my triggers:
- *Tuberous Sclerosis (medical)*
- *Fatigue e.g. late night/early mornings/as I relax down into holiday mode (physiological)*
- *Possibly, hormones e.g. oestrogen (physiological)*
- *Stress e.g. worrying about having more seizures (physiological or environmental)*

Some triggers are uncontrollable such as having TS and fluctuations in hormones, but I can control how much sleep I get and how I can perceive my seizures.

I drew out a diagram highlighting the triggers; followed by the thoughts, feelings, emotions; and then behaviours.

I realise that I'm afraid of being out of control – that I don't want to lose consciousness and I don't know when my next seizure will be. Worrying about the unknown sets me up with more worry. I see a parallel with how I reacted to Anxiety previously.

When I review the second module, I remember that worrying about not knowing what is going to happen is a protective mechanism against danger – perceived or real. The information leaflet in module 2 describes how when we focus on a threat such as a snake, we become more aware of our surroundings – the colour and texture of the snake, where its position is. By looking out for the snake (a real threat if in the jungle) I would less likely be harmed by it.

When I have had an initial seizure, I become more aware of the symptoms I associate with it. I remember the change of smell in the air, the lightheaded sensation and the adrenaline rush that surges down my legs and raises my heartrate. It's not the seizure itself I'm afraid of, but the response my body has after I have had one. If I have a seizure doing an activity such as eating breakfast or watching tv, my hyperawareness of my surroundings comes into play every time I do that activity until I feel it is no longer threatening. If I feel a seizure is threatening, then it intensifies my worry and increases the prospect of a following seizure that has a more intense adrenaline response too. It makes sense why I have previously avoided reading in bed before breakfast as I happen to have an occasional seizure, but neglect to see that more often than not I can read without any seizures happening, just as I have had more breakfasts without having a seizure and watched tv programmes without having a seizure. But I think about those rare times that I have and feel controlled by those few occasions.

"It's not the situation you are in that determines how you feel. It's the thoughts, meanings and interpretations you bring to that situation"
(module 5 – health anxiety clinical interventions)

By module 5, I look at the example from the workbook: Someone hears a noise in the night. They could react to it in a *negative way that someone has broken into their home; they could react in a positive way, that it is probably the cat roaming around; or neutral – that it might be the neighbours' bin outside.*

I think about my epilepsy, and how I can react to an unexpected seizure. Negatively, I think about how another seizure has prevented me from driving for another year, more waiting; filled with disappointment and sadness. However, if I viewed the seizure in a neutral/positive way, I could think I have probably been a bit tired/stressed. Maybe this is a sign to have some self-care and take some time out to relax. I may feel some mild disappointment and concern, but I could still make a note of it in my seizure diary.

By module 7, I review how I can accept vs. control my epilepsy. I note that I take my prescribed medication every day and that I control how much self-care I provide – revisiting getting enough sleep and taking breaks during the day to rest my mind.

I remind myself to accept that epilepsy is a part of my Tuberous Sclerosis and that I may have occasional seizures from time to time that I won't be able to predict or always control.

28th March 2020

I tried too hard yesterday to not have any seizures and I had three over the day. I was revisiting that cycle that my therapist had picked up on that morning – after having one seizure I was afraid of having more. I had to put into practice sitting with that possibility I could have a seizure and be ok with myself if I did.

I decided to watch the next film in the franchise I had watched when I had one of my seizures yesterday. I watched the film with the intent that I may have seizure, almost like allowing a clingy acquaintance to sit next to you even though you would rather ignore them.

The anxiety intensified a bit; some abdominal tension and mild palpations but then the 'clingy acquaintance' settled down a bit and watched the film with me until I was too far lost in the story to think about ignoring the acquaintance any longer.

I felt proud of myself for acknowledging the anxiety and trusting the uncertainty, and I was fine; seizure free as a I normally am when I watch tv. More factual evidence to back-up that watching tv doesn't trigger seizures all the time. With the next film, I put into practice the same skills and I was fine again.

I had started reading a new book this morning; I was fine. I ate breakfast, and I was fine. The activities were the same but my perceptions of them were changing.

As part of accepting my epilepsy, I am realising that this is a process that benefits from repeated practice, just like building a new skill and getting back up when you fall. As I did with Anxiety the first time, I became welcoming of its presence and seeing it not as a threat but a clingy acquaintance that just wants some attention; to know they are cared for, before they can calm down.

Anything a person has ever achieved which is worthwhile, has taken time. For now, my seizures still come and go; at times I get frustrated, disappointed and upset, but then I am reminded about being patient. When I take the pressure off of not having a seizure for a whole year, that urgency dissolves away. I am able to relax, and my brain relaxes. In time, I will be able to drive again.

CHAPTER 2

SKIN, HOW IS IT
AFFECTED BY TSC?

Facial Angiofibromas

One of the most common and external signs that someone might have TSC can be the reddish-pink bumps around their nose and cheeks. The Tuberous Sclerosis Association (TSA) suggests 90% of TSC-affected people have this.

These facial bumps are called Facial Angiofibromas, believed to be an excessive growth of skin tissue caused by an increased presence of blood vessels around those areas: some Facial Angiofibromas showing up in a very prominent way like an angry rash, whilst other people may only have mild skin defects.

Facial Angiofibromas may not be present on an infant at birth but tend to become more noticeable when a child is about five-years-old. The prominence of these facial marks often peaks during adolescence, but there are multiple ways of managing its visibility. For example, as this area of skin is more sensitive to the sun and can become prone to sunburn and increased redness in the heat of a warm day, it is recommended that people with Facial Angiofibromas use sun cream and SPF moisturisers throughout the year to protect their skin.

Other treatments can include a topical cream, involving medication called Sirolimus (also known as Rapamycin) that minimises the growth of the excessive cells, providing a smoother appearance on the skin. However, laser treatment can have a similar effect. This involves a strong wave of light that penetrates the skin and destroys unwanted tissue such as Facial Angiofibromas. Although an effective treatment for some people, others can find it painful and it can cause a regrowth of the original damaged skin.

Hypomelanotic Macules

Although some people with TSC may or may not have the Facial Angiofibromas, 90% may have a white patch of skin on their body called a Hypomelanotic Macule. The shape of these marks is similar to an ash leaf, hence the nickname given by medical professionals. These ash leaf marks are often noticeable at birth and are caused by a lack of melanin that causes our skin and hair to go dark. The levels of melanin are not absent in these patches but just reduced. As with the Facial Angiofibromas, ash leaf marks need extra sun protection.

Shagreen Patches

Around 40% of people with TSC may develop raised flesh-coloured oval bumps on their skin, often found on their lower back. As with the Facial Angiofibromas, these patches are due to an excessive growth of skin and can be found in single locations or in clusters, but don't tend to cause harm. Shagreen Patches provide an external view of how internal organs can be affected by TSC. Similar markings can be found on the brain, kidneys, heart and lungs. If these growths are not monitored and expand in size, then surgery may be needed to treat these areas.

Other skin markings

While the most common skin defects in TSC are illustrated above, other skin conditions may include growths on the nails and raised patches of skin on the forehead. Overall these skin markings don't cause medical issues, but may influence self-esteem, particularly during adolescence.

My Experience

I look down at my knees and try and see where the white patch has gone. It's on one of my knees somewhere but as I have pale skin anyway, it's seemed to have blended in quite well. I remember the ash leaf shaped mark was one of first visual signs that I noticed as my parents told me about TS. This white patch never seemed to be an issue growing up, but for my facial skin, that was different.

Aged twenty-six, I hold two photos in my hand. In the left print, I'm two-years-old, crouched down in the garden, peeping from behind a red and yellow Little Tikes car. In my right hand, two years later, I'm four, this time in a pink ballet leotard and a floral green skirt with a straw hat decorated in flowers made of ribbons; I've just danced to Feed the Birds from Mary Poppins.

When I look at these pictures, it is not so much the toy car or ballet outfit I notice, but how smooth the skin is on my face. When I was four, I was still in the ignorance-is-bliss phase when I wasn't aware that I had TS and neither did my skin. I felt pretty and free.

For a long time, especially during my teens, I would love looking at these prints, longing for that smooth, flawless skin that made me look and feel so happy. I didn't feel pretty as a teenager.

Eurocamp

When I was four turning five, the red, bumpy rash over my nose and cheeks began to form. I wasn't really aware of this until an event on a family holiday in France occurred.

At our campsite I attended a children's day care crèche and I enjoyed having red face paint on and becoming a ladybird. I was playing happily with another girl a few years older than me who had a stripy bee design on her face, and we were having a great time. As the face paint dried, the embossed bumps of my Facial Angiofibromas became more prominent and my new friend told a young male courier in his late teens that she had noticed my skin. I heard the words *allergic reaction* but was confused because I didn't have an allergic reaction to anything. The courier encouraged me to sit down next to the girl, who suddenly became my enemy. I had been happily playing with her and now she was told to keep an eye on me while the courier talked to his colleague. I exchanged awkward glances with the girl while we waited, the temperature in the giant tent stifling me.

The courier came back and encouraged me to follow him out of the tent and along to the row of public toilets. Reluctantly I followed, anger and confusion filling up my whole body. Cold water was then splashed onto my face and the courier briskly wiped off the face paint with a rough paper towel. We returned back to the crèche tent and I was relieved Mum had arrived. I gave her hug and cried all the way back to the tent we were staying in.

That event has been imprinted in my mind ever since that day. At the time I felt I didn't have a say in what was going on and felt judged and ridiculed. In hindsight, I know that the young man had never heard of TS and was reacting with precaution in case the face paint really *was* giving me an allergic reaction. But still, it was a traumatic experience for me.

Childhood

If I wasn't shy already, I became a very self-conscious child after that holiday. I would peep out at the world from under my heavy fringe, Mum says like bit like Princess Diana. On a late Sunday afternoon each member of the family would take turns talking to Granny on the phone and all I would say was "Yep...yep...yep. Bye." Answering the questions Granny would ask me.

I didn't say much in school. It was the bolder, more confident girls who became my friends and as I was yearning for acceptance, I just went along with that they wanted to do. One of my childhood friends, Amy, described me as a bit of mouse but that she found my quietness a relief from the *gaggle of girls* as she described the rest of our class. On parents' evenings teachers explained I was well behaved but often quiet in class, yet I had a loud playground voice.

The playground wasn't all fun though. As my facial skin got redder and bumpier, a group of older girls bullied me for my uneven complexion and those words really cut me to the core. *"Ha ha, look at you! You're all spotty! Ha ha ha!"* I was made to feel ugly as the bullies etched away at what little confidence I had and took advantage of my vulnerable quiet state. Countless times I would cry in my room when I got home, wishing I was like the other girls; not so shy and not so ugly.

Laser treatment/sun cream

When I was about eight-years-old, I was becoming more and more self-conscious of my skin and my parents decided to officially tell me I have TS. I was upset and didn't want to acknowledge the condition; it just seemed unfair that I wasn't like everyone else. Mum and Dad supported me at my TS clinic appointments in Bath. The doctors told us about how they are testing out ways to reduce the inflammation of Facial Angiofibromas. Laser treatment was one option.

We had a consultation with a lady called Cherry Day, and just her name alone made me feel happier and less scared about having a laser beam burning and stinging my skin. I had a few sessions of laser treatment, but for a few days afterwards, my skin looked even worse and more inflamed. When classmates boldly asked me why my skin was red, I lied saying that I fell of my bike. Technically it was true when I was five and I flipped over the handlebars of a bike and scraped my face which appeared in a similar fashion to my lasered skin, but I couldn't bring myself to tell my class the truth. I didn't want to draw more attention than needed. *The laser treatment was supposed to make my skin better, not worse.*

The TS clinic in Bath suggested that I wear sun-cream from at least May to September, to reduce the redness that could be triggered by the ultraviolet rays of the sun.
   "Mum…no one else has to wear sticky sun cream, why do I have to?" I whinged.

Secondary School

The process of adjusting from primary to secondary school was hard, mostly because no other girls or friends from my year were going to my new school and I was lonely. My brown shoulder length hair had grown out, sitting half-way down my back. My heavy, protective fringe now a pair of thick dark curtains, that shielded my face.

Even at eleven, my skin and hair were becoming more and more greasy. As well as my TS facial imperfections, I had real spots regularly forming on my chin, cheeks and forehead. The boys from the popular group would either ignore me or call me spotty, reigniting memories of those primary school days. *They were never going to like me.*

In many ways I felt invisible, spending lunch times alone in the library or clinging to peer groups who either pushed me away or who knew what it was like to be underdogs themselves.

However, a person who saw through my protective barrier of invisibility and greasy curtains from the first day of secondary school was my friend, Molly.

At the end of the taster day I sat on a window seat on the bus, sad and alone, peeping from my curtains. I hadn't made any friends. My day dreaming was interrupted when a girl asked if the seat next to me was taken and if she could sit there. I gave them an awkward smile and a small nod. She boldly introduced herself and I was taken aback at how chatty she was. When I jumped off the bus, Mum was waiting for me. "I've made a friend! I've made a friend!" I beamed.

When we began secondary school officially, Molly and I became regular bus buddies, but as she was in a different tutor group to me, our friendship developed slowly. By Year 8, we would go to each other's houses on a Wednesday and Molly wanted to try out her new eyeshadow kit she had got for her birthday on me. I wrinkled up my face in the discomfort, as she powdered my eyelids. *What if she sees my bumpy skin?*

The following year when we were fourteen, Molly invited me to go to her local youth club with her primary school friend. It was a great place to chat, laugh and have fun after a long day at school. One evening Molly and I were having a tickle fight on the sofa. Red faced and gasping for air, I was full of giggles, I felt a cool draught drifting up my back and yanked my t-shirt down self-consciously. Molly stopped tickling me. "What's that on your back?" she asked curiously. My cheeks flushed now with shame. For a moment there was an awkward silence. In the heavy space, I considered whether to tell her about my condition; I'd never told a friend before. "Come with me," I say, instinctively getting up and encouraging Molly to follow me. We ran out of the back door of the youth club, into the car park and hid behind a wall as the last of the sun was setting. *"Those bumps on my back are to do with a health condition I've got…"*

I didn't go into full detail about TS, but I appreciated that she didn't judge me for having a health condition and felt accepted for who I was.

Experimenting with make-up

Nonetheless I still felt self-conscious of my skin throughout my adolescence and was filled with the discomfort of not having perfect, smooth skin like many girls my age appeared to have. But like them, I began experimenting with make-up and foundation that could minimise the redness of my rash and even out my complexion. I bought some liquid mousse foundation and smoothed it over my skin feeling like a real teenage girl. But when I observed myself in the mirror I was horrified. A monotone screen of pale peach cream sat heavily on my face; the bumps over my nose and cheeks were more pronounced than ever! I hastily wiped the make-up off and chose to go without foundation despite my lack of confidence.

Mum spoke to her friend who worked in a make-up section in a department store. She suggested that if I wanted to take the focus off my skin but still feel pretty, then I could focus on lipstick and eyeshadow instead. I considered this, still slightly haunted by the over-enthusiastic eyeshadow experience at Molly's house.

Mum and I went into the shop and her friend showed me to the chair where I could try on various types of make-up. We tried a soft pink lipstick, neutral brown eyeshadow and mascara. I felt pretty and it definitely improved the appearance of my skin, but I didn't feel like me. Even so, I decided to buy a nude coloured lipstick and the eyeshadow palette.

Throughout the rest of my teens I continued to experiment with the distraction technique. I went through phases where I tried mascara with a black eyeliner pencil along my lower lashes and then going on to just liquid eyeliner along the top. When I got bored of this look, I experimented green liquid eyeshadow at college, before returning to the neutral brown eyeshadow at university and an apple red lip tint. With this look, I felt comfortable.

I revisited foundation again in 2011 when Sarah got married and I tried a powder foundation for my skin, while she tried on wedding dresses. I liked that the powder matched my skin tone and had SPF 15 in it for protection. I bought the powder but as I looked closer in the mirror, I could still see the raised bumps screaming out. I tried the foundation for a few weeks before eventually discarding that look too.

On Sarah's wedding day I asked the make-up artist to apply a natural look, but she began applying gloopy, liquid foundation and I felt like I was wearing a mask. I didn't mind the liner but when I peered into the mirror, I didn't feel like me.

Gaining confidence without a mask

Over the next few years I returned to my neutral brown eyeshadow and mascara, swapping the sticky lip tint for some coral lipstick. The look worked and I felt pretty, but there was something so freeing about the weekend or wandering around an art museum on holiday where I didn't feel the need to wear any make-up. I could just wash my face, get dressed, put on some sun-cream and go about my day; saving the mascara, eyeshadow and lipstick for dressing up at a fancy dinner.

Almost a decade after Sarah's wedding, this mindset began to blend into my everyday world. Who was I wearing this eyeshadow and mascara for? I wasn't getting any satisfaction out of it; rather it seemed like an expectation from society; the norm, and I didn't want to follow that anymore. I wanted to be authentically me. I had the autonomy to be me.

This was at a time I was beginning to acknowledge and accept TS and LAM as something part of me rather than aspects of myself to be ashamed of. With medication slowing the growth of the cysts on my lungs, it was also improving the embossed effect of my Facial Angiofibromas as well. Gradually I experimented without the eyeshadow and just the mascara, before going 100% make-up free, with the exception of special occasions.

Without make-up I feel liberated and genuinely beautiful despite my ever-present flaws.

CHAPTER 3

KIDNEYS, THE TSC AND LYMPHANGIOLEIOMYOMATOSIS (LAM) CONNECTION

What are kidneys?

Kidneys are like filtering systems in our bodies, that are each the size of a clenched fist. They regulate the levels of water and minerals in our bodies, like sodium in our blood and calcium for our bone health. Kidneys also filter blood and toxins that form urine which is removed through the bladder.

Kidneys and Tuberous Sclerosis Complex

The Tuberous Sclerosis Association suggest that 8 out of 10 people with TSC, will have issues with their kidneys. The two common kidney problems connected to the disease are benign tumours called: Renal Cysts and Renal Angiomyolipomas (AMLs).

Renal Cysts

RCs effect 1 in 4 people with TS. The TSA describe RCs to be "present at birth and are like small sack-like lumps of fluid on the kidneys". Most people won't have any issues, but 1 in 20 people may develop many cysts known as polycystic kidneys.

Renal Angiomyolipomas (AMLs)

Renal AMLs are benign tumours that contain fat tissue, abnormal muscle and blood vessels, affecting 8 in 10 people with TS. AMLs begin to develop in childhood and are deemed a safe size until they reach a growth of 4cm. The larger the growth, the more likely the AML will bleed. The TSA suggest that only half the people with AMLs will need any emergency treatment.

How are kidneys monitored for people with TSC?

In my experience below, it was an AML that bled when I was just twenty years old. I used to have ultrasound scans on my kidneys but today myself and others with TSC tend to have our kidneys monitored through either a CT (Computer Tomography) scan or MRI (Magnetic Resonance Imaging) scan. Blood pressure and blood tests also monitor kidney function.

Treatment

If any scans find any abnormal activity, there are several ways in which the patient may be treated. For example, an embolisation uses a metal coil to 'block the blood flow to the tumours' to prevent them from growing. An embolisation is the procedure I had during my AML bleed.

Depending on the situation, treatment may also include medication or a kidney transplant.

TS and LAM

Growths on the kidneys are also connected to the rare lung disease Lymphangioleiomyomatosis (Lim-fan-je-o-li-o-mi-o-ma-to-sis) known as LAM. Although the causes of the condition vary, there is a connection between kidney bleeds, oestrogen and TSC-related LAM. However, just because a person with sporadic LAM has AMLs, doesn't necessarily mean they have TS as well.

My Experience

For as long as I can remember I've been going to the TS clinic at the Royal United Hospital in Bath. On check-up days, I usually had an ultrasound scan. I would lie on the medical table, that was covered in that scratchy greeny/blue paper towelling, with some of it edged around the top of my trousers. Cold, thick, clear jelly was pasted around the sides of my tummy and round my back, and it was always uncomfortable when the fist-shaped scanner pressed against my sides.

Sure, pregnant women were the ones who normally had an ultrasound, but this was routine for me as they monitored my Renal Angiomyolipomas (AMLs). After my scan I would usually have lunch in the hospital café with my parents before going into the main consultation appointment in the children's clinic. As with the MRI scans of my brain being shown up on the computer screen, if I had an ultrasound, we would also look at my kidneys and see how the big the tumours were.

Growing up I was fine, but as I became a teenager, I grew more aware that if the growths were bigger then I had an increased risk of a kidney bleed or surgery; like that would happen.

Subtle Signs

<u>2007</u>

When I was about fourteen, I remember I hadn't used the toilet since I had arrived at school that morning. When I relieved myself, I felt a subtle ache in my side – *woah I really hadn't been to the loo for a few hours.* I acknowledged it, but then dismissed it, as I returned back to my lesson.

2013

In February, I stayed with Geoffrey and his girlfriend while my parents were on holiday. I woke up feeling a groaning ache on my right side. *Maybe I slept in a funny position. Ah well..*

However, before my birthday in the spring, I was dancing in my room and it felt like I had pulled a muscle, but it was near my kidney again. *What is this?*

August 11th 2013

Mum, Dad and I had a bacon sandwich for lunch, busy preparing the house for my relatives who were coming to stay. We are going to Legoland tomorrow.

While my extended family sat in the lounge with Dad, I was slouching on a kitchen chair while Mum was preparing dinner; we were listening to Carly Simon. Suddenly I sneezed. Something shifted in my right side.

After our BBQ and a few drinks, the children were encouraged to go to bed as we have an early start tomorrow. As I climbed into my own bed, I struggled to get to sleep, feeling intense pain increasing in my back and sides.

12th August 2013

I awoke at 6 and drank a glass of orange juice. The pain in my back felt worse and I felt that I could be sick any minute.

As my relatives were waking up, I crept downstairs to Mum and Dad's room, complaining of my sickness, worried about the pain I could feel when I sneezed last night. Mum and Dad tried to calm me down and assured me that I perhaps pulled a muscle.

How could this just be back pain? I was in agony. I rushed to their bathroom and vomited violently several times. As I walked back into their bedroom, everything looked all blurry and my ears were ringing. I felt myself collapse heavily to the floor, just about maintaining some consciousness.

*

Mum and Dad sat me up in their bed. I didn't want breakfast; still feeling sick, the pain so intense. I groaned involuntarily. Is this how painful it is to have a baby and not have a child to hold as a result?

After Mum and Dad phoned the osteopath for an appointment at 10.30, my nine and six-year-old second-cousins overheard that I wouldn't be going to Legoland with them. I felt awful that I couldn't spend time with them. We had all been looking forward to this for months. But I knew that just walking to the lounge with Mum's hot water bottle in my arms was too much of an effort for me.

*

Later that morning, after my extended family continued on to Legoland, I got up from the sofa and felt like I was about to faint again. Mum called urgently to Dad to help me towards the car. I felt so hazy and lightheaded. I was getting weaker by the second.

I decided to keep my head down in the car to stop me from feeling so dreadful, but I still felt so sick. When we got to the osteopath, the practitioner took one look at me and suggested that my parents take me to A&E straight away. The woman gave me a cushion to hold and wished us luck.

*

When we arrived in the hospital, I was just about clinging on to consciousness. Mum and Dad supported me into a wheelchair. We waited in A&E while I got assessed. A medical team came and placed me onto a hospital bed, hooking me up to a machine for a blood transfusion, and water drip to hydrate me – the tests began. I had a cannula in my hand and had my blood pressure taken and some blood tests.

*

The following CT scan revealed the problem was my right kidney and that it was bleeding internally. I then had a two-and-half-hour embolisation operation. I was under local anaesthetic, the kidney area itself being numbed, but I was awake. I drowsily took in my surroundings of a dimly lit, clinical operation room with surgeons around the lower half of my back. Although I couldn't see, they were implanting the metal coil into my kidney to stop it from bleeding. I had lost two-and-a-half pints of blood since last night.

I don't remember much about hospital other than I was continually having tests and my observations done. Mum and Dad took a photo of me in hospital the day after my embolisation, my skin looked yellow. I was anaemic and I didn't want to eat. The chilled food had no flavour and I just felt dreadful.

2nd September 2013

Today I had a doctor's appointment. Mum and I went along. My haemoglobin levels (my red blood cell count) were 9.6 and needed to be 12 – a level of 75% oxygen in my blood. I was prescribed iron tablets for the following six weeks and to eat as much calorific food as I could. I had lost 3 stone and was weighing below 7. Mars bars and fizzy drinks have not been my usual diet, especially since I was cutting unhealthy treats out to help with my health anxiety. I had avoided becoming unwell, but I still did anyway.

September 5ᵗʰ 2013

Recovery presents itself with various obstacles and road bumps even after the fall. It's about getting up and trying again; knowing when to rest and when to play, but not push too far. Life presents itself with the unexpected. I wasn't imagining I would have a kidney bleed in August or imagine my stomach misbehaving. I just want to be more mobile.

9ᵗʰ September 2013

Mum and Dad took me outside to get some air into my lungs whilst I'm being stuck indoors all day. They took me to town and got me hot chocolate with whipped cream. I managed to hobble around the top level of the shopping centre, hooking my arm around Dad's for support.

12ᵗʰ September 2013

It's a month ago since the bleed. I never realised how busy I was until I became ill. My mind is feeling more active now, but my body isn't feeling up to what it was used to. I was trying to make everything so perfect but now I'm accepting that I can only go so far before I get tired again. I'm better when I know my limits.

13ᵗʰ September 2013

Managed a walk around the block today with Mum. I felt a little wobbly and faint as went up the gentle hill, but as the pavement became even, I felt less dizzy and more able to do it. I'm learning to listen to my body more. Decided to have a rest in the afternoon and feel grateful for that.

22ⁿᵈ September 2013

I'm so glad I was able to go to our local agricultural show today. It is one of my favourite days of the year and I was able to enjoy it in a wheelchair Mum and Dad hired. I loved watching the horses show-jumping and I bought a red rosette in the craft tent. I had never got one while I used to go horse-riding, but this real-life achievement was way more important than winning a competition at a riding school. I had been through a kidney bleed and I was recovering. I deserve this rosette!

29th September 2013

I just feel so negative right now. My confidence is low, and I've got university coursework to do. I'm just so stressed. I spent all those months doing my CBT therapy, then I was ill and now I'm anxious again. Life is so overwhelming!

October 12th 2013

Today I went on an autumnal sensory walk around the village. It's been so nice living back at home and enjoying the countryside again. I picked conkers with mum and inhaled the fresh cool air. I'm getting better at pacing myself with my walking and stamina. If I have learnt anything from being ill, it is pace and slowing down to listen to your body.

October 18th 2013

I think my haemoglobin levels are still low as I almost fainted having my blood test done, and I was lying down. It took me back to That Day.

October 21st 2013

Rest is important. These couple of days, although frustrating at times, have been teaching me how my body needs to recover so that it can repair itself. Sometimes my only option is to lie down and I'm facing and learning about the emotional and physical discomfort I tried to avoid before I had therapy and before I was unwell. By learning this now, I need to carry it on, even when I feel better, and not take advantage of my abilities; taking breaks in between tasks like my coursework and setting aside time to do fun activities.

October 28th 2013

Good and wonderful news! I'M NO LONGER ANAEMIC! It is such a great feeling! 12.8 is within the normal haemoglobin range and before it was 9.6. I still had some way to go but I'm so excited!

I managed my energy levels closely today and took a break from my coursework in the morning, one for lunch and one in the afternoon as well. With that burst of energy, I took some impromptu photos in the garden.

I've been on two walks this past week and I had energy left to spare!

November 15th 2013

I enjoyed having a cup of tea at my neighbour's house this afternoon. The elderly couple said I was looking well. Betty grabbed her camera, taking a picture of me, telling me I looked so nice. That was really heart-warming to hear. Looking at the photo, I can really see the colour in my cheeks, compared to the photo Mum and Dad took of me the day after my embolisation. I take that as a good sign that I'm looking and feeling better.

This evening we watched Children in Need. It was extremely emotional considering what I have been through this year. There was a hospice for children called "Zoë's Place" and the girl in the film, who lost her brother, was called Zoë. When the video clip ended, Terry Wogan said to the camera "You are a very brave girl, Zoë."

Even though he wasn't speaking directly to me, I pretended he was. I silently thanked Terry, and Mum then said to us: "We have our own very brave Zoë here." And the three of us cried together.

November 25th 2013

Today I had a check-up in Bath. We arrived just before 9 and I had my ultrasound done by the same lady who had done it previously. I felt myself tense up when the scanner gently prodded my right side; if it felt sensitive in the past, it felt even more sensitive now, especially near my ribs where I had lost weight.

After the scan I stood on the weighing scales; I had put on 2 stone since August, weighing 8st 12. Just another stone to go before I was back to my usual weight.

In my consultation, my parents spoke of their concern about my low energy levels. I tried to assure them I was ok, and it was part of my recovery. Dr Amin confirmed that while my red blood cell count may be good, the iron levels in my blood may still be low, which may be why I still get tired from time to time. I was relieved but also disappointed that I still had some more recovering to do.

*

20th August 2014

I think it was a year ago today that I came out of hospital. It felt like Christmas! I was happy to be home and spent the next few months in Sarah's spacious old bedroom with the big double bed all to myself. Dad had made his egg-battered fish with some veg. Wow! That rich tasting meal was way better than the hospital food!

If I had wondered what I would have done within a year, I would have been surprised. I completed my CBT therapy for anxiety, created a motivation board for my room; got my BA (hons) degree in Photography; turned 21; and completed a 7-mile walk in the countryside with Mum.

*That 7-mile walk was proof that I was better. I am better!
We had a picnic and an ice-cream and when we got home,
I celebrated with my 'Well done Zoë' mug that I got after my
degree. Life is looking better.*

Although I didn't know it at the time, as I was entering my
twenties, my oestrogen levels were rising. I was told that this
rise in oestrogen most likely triggered my kidney bleed, and
was a possible factor towards developing Tuberous Sclerosis
related LAM.

Five years later, after my kidney bleed, the size of my AML
had decreased due to the success of the operation. I also found
the courage to go to Legoland when I had been so afraid to.
I was scared of the theme park, but then I remembered I never
got there on that horrible day. I realised that it was my
association of the event that I had connected to Legoland,
which stopped me from going. To go to Legoland in 2018 was
a wonderful experience.

CHAPTER 4

LUNGS AND LYMPHANGIOLEIMYOMATOSIS (LAM)

What is LAM?

Lymphangioleimyomatosis (LAM) is a rare lung disease related to Tuberous Sclerosis Complex (TSC). While 1 in 6,000 people have TSC, 7 in 1 million have either the sporadic or TSC-related LAM. In the UK alone, under 500 women are currently diagnosed.

LAM Action, one of the leading UK charities describes what makes the term Lymphangioleimyomatosis:

"The name Lymphangioleiomyomatosis reflects the different components of the disease. Lymph and angio refer to the lymph and blood vessels that are involved and leiomyo refers to smooth muscle which LAM cells resemble."

(LAM Action)

As with TSC, this lung condition involves the same set of faulty genes – TSC1 and TSC2. LAM cells can grow inside the lungs, around the lymph and blood vessels, as well as the respiratory airways. *LAM Action* describes that the lymph vessels drain excess fluid from the lungs and that LAM cells can develop into cysts which replace normal lung tissue.

Like those who have Tuberous Sclerosis Complex, people with stand-alone sporadic LAM may have the similar growths on their kidneys called Angiomyolipomas (AMLs). These kidney tumours may vary in size but can potentially bleed and would need urgent medical attention.

Early Signs of LAM

Due to connections with the female hormone oestrogen, women are most likely to be affected by LAM. This in turn can cause the condition to develop when a woman reaches child-bearing age, such as in her early twenties when her oestrogen levels rise. Although research is still taking place, it is possible that the increased hormone level can spur the growth of the LAM cells, which may have been dormant throughout childhood and adolescence.

Although shortness of breath may be associated with other respiratory conditions such as Asthma and Chronic Obstructive Pulmonary Disease (COPD), breathlessness in LAM could potentially mean that a large area of the lung is covered in cysts which makes breathing a daily struggle, or that a lung cyst may have burst, causing the lung to collapse. The medical name for this is called a Spontaneous Pneumothorax, which often accompanies the breathlessness with sharp shoulder pain and would need immediate medical attention.

If the air leak is small, a special tool, known as a chest drain, can draw out excess air that had escaped to inflate the lung. If there was a large lung collapse or a person had experienced multiple pneumothoraces, then a medical procedure called a pleurodesis can help attach the lung to the chest wall to prevent further collapses.

Not everyone with LAM will experience a pneumothorax, but as it's a progressive disease, they will more likely occur if a person is unaware they have the condition.

Other complications

Like TSC, LAM can vary from person to person. Some women may have a mild form of the disease that has minimal impact on their lives whereas others may find that LAM is deteriorating their lung health a lot faster.

In the past women may have only discovered they had LAM upon needing a lung transplant or requiring portable oxygen cylinders, but this is far less common today thanks to technology and research. While Magnetic Resonance Imaging (MRI) scans may be able to show tumours in organs such as the brain and kidneys, LAM cells are harder to identify. CT scans, known as Computerised Tomography, can scan for higher quality images of inside the body, which can identify LAM related cysts. Regular scans can help monitor any changes in the size of cysts over time.

Often individuals may discover they have LAM from the changes in hormones, such as when reaching child-bearing age or during pregnancy, that may have caused a lung to collapse. In some cases, women who already have a LAM diagnosis may be medically advised not to get pregnant as their lung health could become unstable with the increased levels of oestrogen. Changes in air pressure when flying in an aeroplane may also present itself with issues, so if there are any concerns, it is good to check with your doctor or LAM specialist first.

The UK National LAM Centre

As LAM is such a rare disease many medical professionals have not even heard of it. However, in April 2011, Professor Simon Johnson, an expert in respiratory medicine who had completed research into the disease, set up the UK National LAM Centre at the Queen's Medical Centre, part of the Nottingham University Hospitals NHS Trust.

The National LAM Centre helps to monitor patients with both sporadic and TSC-related versions of LAM and to support the diagnosis process with the patient's local doctor. To monitor the lung health of someone with LAM, pulmonary tests are used to measure lung function. These series of tests show how well the lungs work, including how much oxygen is transferred into the patient's bloodstream after they have inhaled and exhaled all the way out to their full capacity. For example, regular monitoring can illustrate how well the lungs are working, such as showing the difference in lung function before and after surgery.

Treatment

Although there is yet to be a cure for LAM or Tuberous Sclerosis Complex, a medicine called Rapamycin/Sirolimus can help both conditions. It helps to reduce the size of kidney AMLs and preserve healthier lung function, as well as minimising the size of tumours in the brain and skin lesions in TSC.

LAM Action Charity

Alongside the National LAM Centre, the UK charity LAM Action, was set up in 2003. The charity helps to raise money and awareness of the disease, as well as supporting people with LAM. Updates on medical research and charity events are published within a newsletter called LAM Post, which women with LAM can contribute to. What started with 21 people, LAM Action now has over 150 members, many of whom meet up in regional areas of the country.

For further details on LAM Action, the National LAM Centre, as well as links to organisations around the world, visit: http://lamaction.org

My Experiences

When I was about eleven, I remember seeing a poster about LAM in the TS clinic in Bath. The disease sounded really scary and something I didn't want to have. I didn't know at the time, that it would be something I would develop within the next decade.

November 2011

In September I began the first year of my photography degree at the University of West London. I was eighteen and it was great opportunity to meet lots of creative people and five of us developed a nice little a friendship group.

In November, we had an opportunity to go on a photography trip to Prague. With winter almost coming, it was cold, and we could hardly see past the end of our noses with so much fog surrounding us.

Over the autumn I had developed a nasty cough, which I took to Prague with me. After a week of taking photos, going to night clubs and drinking lots of alcohol, I returned home, my cough even more phlegmy, making me feel really unwell. By the end of the week the cough got worse and my parents were on holiday. On the Friday night home alone, I had a life-threatening choking episode.

19th November 2011

This morning I woke up in the spare room of my neighbour's house. Last night was really scary. With Mum and Dad on holiday in Iceland, I remembered having Spaghetti Bolognese in front of the tv at home. As I swallowed my food, I needed to cough, but it was like my tummy couldn't take anymore food in and I felt an acidic-food mixture come up back up. The acid taste tickled the back of my throat and the bile took a detour down my windpipe. I tried to clear my airways, but no sound was coming out. I tried to cough again. Silence.

With only the air in my lungs keeping me alive and conscious, I rushed to the front door and unlocked it, closed it behind me and ran across the road to my neighbour's house. I knocked frantically at the door, still with no sound or breath coming out of my airways. I was possibly inches away from suffocating.

Betty opened the door. I pointed hysterically at my throat and my back. Betty let me in and said to her husband, Eric, that I'm choking. Betty used to be nurse when she was younger, but I didn't know this at the time.

Rather than patting me on my back, Betty firmly patted the sides of my ribs with both hands. Still no sound was coming out of my mouth. After more patting, eventually, I was able to take a breath in and vomited the food, blood and phlegm from my lungs into a bucket.

Eric and Betty agreed it was best if I stayed with them that night. Betty gave me plenty of water and helped calm me down. My airways went into spasm and I was croaking with the croup I had developed, yet I managed to get a restful sleep.

Eric and Betty treated me to a pub lunch and said they had told my parents what had happened the night before. They were on their way back from Iceland.

The following week, my cough was still playing up and I went to the doctor's with Mum. Dr Keast listened to my chest and told us that I had Bronchitis. It was frustrating to hear but also a relief to put a name to why I had been feeling so horrible. I was given a temporary inhaler to help me breathe.

2012

This year was better; my Bronchitis had cleared up and I enjoyed watching the London 2012 Olympics and the Paralympics in the summer. In the autumn I began my second year of university and moved into student accommodation.

4th December 2012

Although I enjoyed coming home for the weekend to decorate the Christmas tree, I did have a bit of a scare.

On Friday, Mum and Dad picked me up from London and we bought our Christmas tree on the way home. The next morning, we put on some Christmas music and I danced wildly around the lounge as they got the decorations down from the loft.

Dad put the fairy lights on the tree first and then I got some tinsel, raising my arms up to reach the tallest branches. As I reached up, I felt a sharp pull in my chest and in my left shoulder. It was like the muscles around my shoulder seized up and it was becoming more and more painful. I tried sitting on the sofa to relax, but my shoulder and chest felt so sore.

Mum and Dad suggested I lie down on the fluffy rug just to relieve my muscles. After a few moments I felt better and got up, continuing to decorate the tree and enjoying the music.

The following morning, I woke up my chest muscles still feeling tense. I also noticed that I felt out of breath. I went downstairs to tell Mum and Dad that I was worried. When I mentioned chest pain and shortness of breath, they decided to call 111.

As it was a Sunday, we couldn't just pop down the doctor's to see what was wrong. Before we had breakfast, the on-call ambulance service a few miles away came immediately. I was briskly wired up to an ECG machine to monitor the rhythm and speed of my heart. Given an ok on that, I had a clip attached to my finger to monitor my oxygen levels. All good. Next I had my blood pressure checked and my chest listened to.

We were told by the ambulance staff that I would be ok within a week, and that my chest muscles had probably gone into *spasm when I was decorating the tree. I was given some shoulder exercises to do.*

*

It's been some weekend. I have just got back to my student flat in London and my shoulder is still sensitive. At least my health is all right, but it's been really emotional.

Throughout the Christmas period I continued my exercises and life seemed to be returning to normal.

2013

In May, Sarah gave birth to my eldest nephew. I really enjoyed becoming an Auntie and spent a lot of time with him while I was recovering from my kidney bleed that summer. As I grew stronger, I began to pick him up, pushing him on the swings in the playpark.

2014

By the following summer, I had graduated from university and my little nephew was learning to walk. On the days my parents and I looked after him, we took him out for the day.

16th September 2014

Today we went to a National Trust house and had a picnic. We had sandwiches and crisps. Dad had a nap on the picnic blanket while Mum and I ran around after my nephew until we were chasing the smell of his nappy. Mum sorted out the changing mat and I went to down to pick up him. But as I did, I could hear a crack, and felt something pull and click around my ribs. It was really painful.

19th September 2014

My chest still feels a bit sore from the other day, but it's my shoulder that is really hurting. Today I went to the Osteopath who checked over my back and suggested doing some yoga to help strengthen my shoulders.

21st September 2014

I went to a yoga class today. Usually I find it relaxing, but as I was balancing my weight on my arms doing a Downward-Facing-Dog, my shoulder felt really sensitive. It was a shame I couldn't enjoy it.

At least I had the local country show to look forward to. Last year I was in a wheelchair, but this year I could walk around… for most of it anyway. I enjoyed all the stalls and the horses, but I felt drained by the end of the day. When we walked back to Dad's truck, my lungs felt really heavy and the air seemed really thick. My shoulder still hurts.

24th September 2014

My breathing felt better when I went to town with Mum. Today, I went to the job centre and although the interview seemed to go well, my chest felt all constricted again like it did at the country show. Dad thinks that my muscles have probably gone into spasm again like they did two years ago. Mum booked an appointment at the doctor's tomorrow. She is encouraging me to walk there to show how unusually out of breath I am. I really don't want to do this. I wish she knew how much hard work it will be.

25th September 2014

With my state worsening, Dad agreed that he would drive me to the doctor's. I was coughing and wheezing as I ambled from the car to the surgery. Dr Keast listened to my chest. Apparently, shortness of breath and shoulder pain means one of my lungs has collapsed. He was 100% sure it was a Pneumothorax not shoulder pain.

Dad drove me to casualty, and we were told we were in for a long night of tests.

*

"Ok, Zoë, we have detected the problem and you have what is called a spontaneous pneumothorax. How this works is by air leaking from your lung that has gathered around the chest wall putting pressure on your lung, which made it collapse. Luckily, we can still do something about it, so if is ok, we're going insert a chest drain into you, that will help remove the excess air and help your lung inflate again."

Throughout the conversation I simply nodded and accepted it because I wanted this all to be over. Once the procedure was explained, I was to sit on the edge of the bed hunched over two pillows so that my shoulder was exposed. I tried to sit comfortably but it was challenging for twenty minutes.

First off was the anaesthetic which numbed the area where it would be safe to insert a chest drain. The anaesthetic stung like crazy but was nothing to the thick tube being inserted between my ribs into my chest wall. The pain whizzed round my shoulder, as the tube got deeper inside my chest. It was agonising.

When it was in, I could sit up. The dizziness from the pain subsided and I looked up at Dad and the medical team. Looking down my left side I spotted the chest drain tube was connected to a bucket with clear liquid at the bottom that bubbled as the excess air from my lung flowed in. I would need this until my lung was fully healed. Although still in pain my blood pressure dropped to a reasonable 130 and my oxygen level was now 100, with the help of the drain.

RARE: A JOURNEY OF SELF-ACCEPTANCE

Mum had arrived after my procedure and it was now reaching 10pm. A bed was waiting for me in the thoracic ward where I was wheeled through the hospital. Somehow, I would have to transfer from one bed to another. I thought back to how I did this after my kidney embolisation, using a hard board used for transferring safely, if not comfortably.

This time was just as excruciating to transfer and the searing pain in my side caused me to cough, the chest drain rattling inside me. My throat was tickly and I was gagging, crying and panicking at the same time. I practiced breathing deeply the best I could, and the coughing eased off. I was in need of a good night's sleep.

26th September 2014

I could feel the chest drain tube move between my ribs as I inhaled and exhaled. In my wakeful hours last night I realised my lung must have collapsed ten days ago when I picked up my nephew at the National Trust house. I had no idea this was going to happen.

*

Sarah came to visit today. She brought me a big cuddly toy to cheer me up, while Mum and Dad took turns visiting me and spending time in the hospital café before going home at night.

September 28th 2014

It's not nice having lots of injections and tests. Each day I have some blood thinner injected into my tummy to help with my circulation.

I'm learning that it takes time for lungs to heal after a Pneumothorax. Some people need a chest drain, some don't. It makes me wonder whether that time I was decorating the Christmas tree was a small Pneumothorax that healed by itself. Chest and shoulder pain - highly likely.

The doctors are saying it could be a couple more days before my lung starts to inflate. As it had collapsed so much – I imagine like a deflated balloon – the team have connected my chest drain to a suction machine to help it inflate faster.

The following day, I was transferred by ambulance to Guy's Hospital in London. I was due to have an operation where a metal clip would be inserted into the top of my lung to hold it up. The operation was delayed due to another patient needing a lung transplant. I waited the next day, and the next, getting bored of being 'nil by mouth'.

Eventually when my operation was confirmed, I eagerly climbed onto the trolley that would take me to the operating room. I had my procedure midday and came out of Recovery in the evening.

The staff at Guy's kept an eye on me and my parents visited regularly. I had a chest x-ray every day and my dressings changed, but every time the staff tried to replace my chest drain, my lung kept collapsing slightly, despite the metal clip.

The medical team decided to do a Pleurodesis to help the lung stick once and for all. On this occasion, they took a syringe of blood from my arm and injected it into the side of my ribs, to irritate the chest wall, so the lung would stick.

It was during this time at Guy's that I found out I had LAM. When I thought back to that poster I saw in Bath all those years ago, I never thought I would be relieved to find out I had it. I was just so pleased it wasn't anything worse. The connection to TS made LAM seem familiar, so in a way, I was grateful to finally have a diagnosis. I was sent home with a chest drain, a few days later.

October 20th 2014

It was an early start to go to Guy's, as an outpatient this morning. I had an x-ray; my dressings changed and had a fresh chest drain put in. I wish my thinking was more positive. I worry something worse will happen to me. I know it's not guaranteed, but I'm scared. I just need to be positive. I hope things get better.

October 24th 2014

Today I did some colouring in the kitchen and it is really helping with my low mood. Mum and I tried a walk today. We walked slowly, pausing for a breath, admiring the countryside view from the benches we paused on. I'm pleased I was able to walk about half a mile.

3rd November 2014

Another outpatient's appointment at Guy's. I met the man who did my surgery and he gave me the choice on how long I wanted to keep the chest drain in for. I decided to have it in for another two weeks.

Throughout that time, I had more check-ups and more dressing changes. In my next follow-up at Guy's, my lung had mostly stuck to my chest wall, but I may need another operation for it to fully stick. It was disappointing, but nothing new. I just wanted to be well again.

21st November 2014

It was nice when the thoracic team greeted me on my return to their ward yesterday.
This morning I had a blood test and I signed the consent form for my surgery. In the afternoon I had my op.

I remember the cold, burning liquid going into my hand as I went under general anaesthetic. The Pleurodesis was just under an hour, but rather than using my blood to irritate the chest wall, they used talcum powder, a common alternative.

For the next week I waited in hospital while my lung began to attach itself to my chest. On the 26th my chest x-ray showed that my lung had dropped a little bit and they took a clamp off my chest drain to help it re-inflate.

While I was in hospital, I did some exercises in the thoracic gym to improve my lung capacity: 5 minutes walking on the treadmill, 10 minutes on the exercise bike in the morning, and the reverse in the afternoon.

27th November 2014

Good news! I have had the chest drain out! Having it removed was a bit like giving birth to an umbilical cord through my ribs as well as a Genie who has been freed from his lamp. My breathing seems good and I'm breathing my own air! I'm doing it myself!

I've been told that my lung has sealed nicely to my chest wall, but there're is a slight gap of air at the top. The doctor assured me that with exercise, the air pocket will heal up on its own.

30th November 2014

My throat feels tight. I had 3 x-rays that have shown me I'm fine, so why am I worrying so much? It's these 24 hours after being discharged that scare me. What if I have go back into hospital? What if I can't breathe? I'm so conscious about all the aches and pains I have felt, that I can't stop thinking about them. It's been a long journey. My shoulder feels a bit sore. It's probably all part of the recovery.

I feel better from having a cry. It's helped to release some of that tension I've been feeling. I've got to trust myself that my lungs can help me breathe and that I am ok.

As December came around, I enjoyed listening to the Christmas music, while I watched Mum and Dad decorate the tree. My body still ached, and I felt tired, pleased that I could have my stitches removed just before Christmas.

2015

Life was looking more positive as I entered 2015. I was recovering from my surgery, but I could begin focusing on getting a job and starting my counselling training.

In February my parents and I accepted a visit to the National LAM Centre in Nottingham. I had my first lung function test and a check-up with Professor Johnson. The lung function test was quite hard as I still felt very protective of my lungs and breathing in, to my fullest capacity and then out, was really difficult. My lung function was a little on the low side, but I had recently had an operation.

Professor Johnson told us that I have TS-related LAM. He explained the connection between LAM and the Pneumothoraces, and 80% of women with TS develop cysts on the lungs and kidneys in early adulthood. It made sense why I had my kidney bled when I was twenty and I had issues with my lungs aged twenty-one.

It was sad to hear that in order to protect my health, Professor Johnson medically advised me not to get pregnant naturally when I decide to have children. It was hard news to accept because other than LAM, there was no reason why my body wouldn't be able to produce a child. But after hearing how undiagnosed pregnant women with LAM have lung collapses, I could see that it may not be a good idea for me or an unborn baby. At that time, I wanted to curse my oestrogen, but I realised that this hormone makes me a woman and that makes me – me.

On that day in February, I also learnt that flying in an aeroplane may cause some risk to my lungs. Another hard pill to swallow as I have travelled on a plane may times throughout my life. I thought about the first holiday in Canada at less than a year old; being seven in the year 2000 at sunny Disney World, Florida; and spending my twelfth birthday in some of the most famous cities on West Coast of America. Was I ever going to see those places again?

By March I was getting more job interviews and I successfully made the second round of a Support Worker role at Mencap. I jumped up and down with joy but then my right shoulder began to hurt. I wasn't breathless, so I assured myself I was fine.

The following day I had my hair cut and my hairdresser said I was looking well. That to me proved I was ok. But as I walked home, I had a slight wheeze to my breath. *This could not be happening to me again.*

1st *April 2015*

Mum and Dad were out when I got home. I took my things upstairs and sat on my bed, letting warm tears slide down my face. I made myself some soup for lunch and waited for Molly to come round. She hugged me when she arrived, but I could tell something in my chest didn't feel right. When we walked up the stairs, I noticed how breathless I was feeling. Even talking to her, my lungs were struggling for air.

I excused myself, saying I just needed to get some paracetamol from downstairs, and then I phoned Mum. After I hung up, I explained to Molly what I thought was wrong and we sat silently on my bed as she held my hand in hers.

*

Mum called the doctor's and got an access appointment for me in the mid-afternoon. Molly waited to be picked up.

At the doctor's I explained that I was breathless, and my right shoulder was hurting. Dr Keast mulled over how it was my shoulder that hurt last time. He listened to my chest and said he could hear the air in my lungs going to all the right places. Nonetheless he suggested I have a chest x-ray at A&E just in case.

*

Mum drove to me the hospital as I clutched the letters detailing all my TS/LAM information; my chest heaving as I sobbed all the way there.

When we got to the hospital, I asked Mum if I could have wheelchair. She wheeled me to A&E and bypassed triage as we already had the documents. After the x-ray I was shocked to find out that I had two Pneumothoraces. *How could this be possible?*

Mum explained to the x-ray team that my left lung shouldn't have collapsed due to the multiple operations I had on it. They phoned Guy's Hospital to ask for their opinion. We discovered that there was still a slight gap at the top of my left lung, but it was stable. However, I did have an air leak on my right lung.

April 1st 2015 (continued)

This was becoming a familiar process to me. I was stripped out of my clothes into a green gown and team of nurses and doctors inserted a needle to get some blood. I was frozen –not from the shock but shivering due to a lack of clothing. My oxygen was no longer 100, but 89. I had an oxygen mask put over my nose and mouth.

There was so much activity around me as the hospital staff rushed around. A thin needle was inserted into the right side of my chest to suck out the excess air around my chest wall and my lung gradually re-inflated.

April 2nd 2015

I spent last night in the high intensity ward and was moved to another ward this afternoon. Izzy came to visit, and I explained to her all about TS/LAM and how oestrogen is big issue at the moment. It was great to have a friend around for support.

April 3rd 2015

Mum and Dad had popped home last night and came into today with my pjs, dressing gown and a hot cross bun. Although I still had my oxygen mask, I was able to go down from 10ml of Oxygen to 5ml, so hopefully that means my lung is getting stronger.

April 5th 2015

It's Easter! Mum, Dad and Geoffrey have just been to visit Sarah and her family. Mum showed me a video on her phone of them saying "Happy Easter!" to me. Geoff gave me a mint chocolate Easter egg.

The weekend doctor came around to check on the patients in the ward. He said to me that if my x-ray looks good today, then I would be able to go home tomorrow. That would be fantastic!

After my x-ray the doctor contacted Guy's Hospital, asking whether I should have a planned pleurodesis on my right lung, just so it doesn't collapse again. I sighed knowing that I didn't want to go through more collapses, if I could avoid it.

April 6th 2015

I will have to wait until I know the date of my operation, but for now I've been told that I can go home. There is still a small leak on the right side, but I'm making good progress. I've got to come in next week for another chest x-ray and been advised to take it easy. I probably will have to defer my upcoming job interview as well.

It was great to back home. I spent the next couple of days resting on the sun-lounger in my pyjamas enjoying the spring weather. The following Sunday, we had a delayed Easter and pre-birthday celebration with the family; them finding Easter eggs and me receiving presents.

My twenty-second birthday was a lovely sunny day. I had a pub lunch with Mum and Dad, a refreshing shower and opened the rest of my presents.

17th April 2015

My shoulders are tense especially my right one. I just hope I will be all right until my op. It was hard finding out yesterday when my operation is going to be. As I write, my stomach is clenching, and my hand is shaking.

23rd April 2015

It's one week until operation day. I just feel like one wrong move and I will snap in two. Feeling very insecure right now and so bothered about what the doctors said about taking it easy. I AM taking it easy! But I feel so limited in what I can do.

Despite not knowing if I was able to even attend my Mencap interview the following day, I managed to go and luckily was offered the job, there and then. It was fantastic news during such a turbulent time. I allowed myself to really feel happy, and that I really deserved this role. Finally, employment!

29th April 2015

Mum and Dad brought me to Guy's Hospital as it was admission day. It was funny when one of the nurses said:

"Zoë, what are you doing back here?" but it felt nice to be recognised and welcomed back to the ward.

At 9pm I had my observations done and despite having an operation tomorrow, my blood pressure was surprisingly relaxed.

After the nurse left, I pulled my curtain across and gazed out the window. It is like having my own private view of the London skyline at night. I can see the blue lights on the London Eye against the purple sky; a complete contrast to the black, starry sky back at home.

The following day, my right lung Pleurodesis was a success. By the afternoon, my lung was already beginning to stick to my chest.

May

I was doing well with my breathing while I was resting most of the day in my hospital bed, but when I had my chest drain removed and began to walk around, I became breathless. A nurse took a blood test and listened to my chest – she said I was fine. The next day, a doctor suggested I have an x-ray and to go back onto a chest drain. Mum looked worried, tears forming in her eyes. I felt numb with emotion.

Over the next few days, I had created a plan with the thoracic ward managers about exercises I could do to help my lungs. Every two hours I would do some breathing exercises and, in the hours, in between I would do 10 minutes walking in the thoracic gym.

11th May 2015

My exercise regime had been going so well...or so I thought. The doctors came round to say that I will need another *pleurodesis as my chest drain had stopped working. It's not fair!*

Over the next couple of days my mind was a blur. I had another chest drain inserted higher up my rib cage in order to help the last bit of lung to stick to my chest wall; more tests, and more feelings of sickness due to nerves.

13th May 2015

If I was going to be sick, I did not want it to go into my lungs like I did on that dark November night. I'm scared the talcum powder won't work. This time I was awake, under local anaesthetic.

3 syringes were inserted with some water to dilute the talc so it would harden against the chest wall. I felt like I was upside down. I let out a loud cry, tears burning my eyes.

"You can cry, Zoë, all you want," – said Mum by my bed, as I howled and howled.

For the next two hours, Mum stayed by me while the Pleurodesis worked its magic. I hugged a folded towel over my stomach, allowing myself to breathe deeply and calm myself down. Eventually I closed my eyes was able to rest.

14th May 2015

I'm on suction today, just to make sure my lung is staying up. The surgeon who did my pleurodesis said I tolerated the procedure better than most. That felt like a real compliment, considering what I have been through.

15th May 2015

I feel so much better after a deep sleep. My breathing feels a little tight on my right side and I was little breathless after exercise, but my appetite is better. I ate some cornflakes and drank some orange juice.

17th May 2015

Just been told by the doctor that from my last x-ray he has noticed that there isn't air leak or excess drainage coming from my lung. This is fantastic! I'm so happy! He informed me that they are taking things slowly so they won't take my chest drain out yet, but I'm making good progress.

Two days later, I had my chest drain removed. The doctor recommended they kept me in one more night to make sure the lung would still stay up without the drain. After one more chest x-ray, the following morning, I was able finally to go home.

As I had one more walk around the ward and the gym, I passed lots of staff that I had got to know over the last few months. Some nurses were sad to see me go; others wished me luck on my way. *"You've been a good patient"*, said the doctor.

Recovery

There many different ways to describe the word *recovery*. The Cambridge Dictionary describes recovery as in getting better after an illness, but that only provides a small meaning to the experiences I faced. Another definition that they give which best describes my recovery is:

> *"a process in which a situation improves after a difficult period"*
>
> Cambridge Dictionary

It took a while until I began feeling like myself. When I first came out of hospital, I was sitting on my bed for long periods of time; sleeping, staring out of the window, reading and listening to music. I was bored. My sides felt sore and I couldn't face looking at my wounds in the mirror for a long time.

29th May 2015

Mum says, "I'm brave. An example to us all"

I'm brave because of what I have been through, but I had no choice. I know that having those procedures would make me better in the long run. People think that being brave is not about being scared, but actually it's about taking that giant step, despite feeling afraid. If someone says I'm brave for what I have experienced, then I can agree. I don't feel it's something I need to show off about, but it's a quiet achievement for myself. I had the last remaining stitches removed today.

A month later I had my last follow up appointment at my local hospital. I was told that my lungs are stable, but it's important that I still don't fly in a plane. It was a bit disappointing, but I didn't feel ready to anyway. I knew that I was going to have to keep an eye on my body and make sure that I look after it well.

27th June 2015

I don't want to be afraid of my body. I know it will take some time. I'm worried about my oestrogen. I'm using those old avoidance techniques to numb out any negativity. Deep down I know the best thing for me to do is to accept my feelings.

25th July 2015

It's occurred to me how much I need to trust myself. To trust my body after traumatic experiences. That I can only control what I can and accept what I can't.

I knew I could control how much exercise I was doing for my body, as I needed to build up my lung capacity. I began with walking up and down the stairs at home, but I kept getting breathless. I walked on the level ground in the garden; that was better. I looked online for ways to increase lung capacity and tried some singing.

I began with *Twinkle, Twinkle Little Star,* but just saying the words out loud were making me breathless. Then I tried some breathing exercises; inhaling all the way in and exhaling all the way out, my chest wall felt sore. I found some old singing exam warm-up clips from several years ago; lots of "ooooh's and aaahs" – that was helpful. But slow. Progress seemed very slow.

But the more I practised singing and pushed the distances that I would walk, my lung capacity began to stretch, and my breathing improved.

In August, we went on a family holiday for Dad's birthday. I had read that swimming was good for lung capacity, but as I jumped in and tried to doggy paddle, my lungs felt like heavy iron buoys inside my chest, being dragged along the water. This confirmed that my lungs were firmly stuck to my chest wall, but the shock from not knowing how swimming would feel was terrifying and really discouraging. *How was I going to use swimming now to help with my lung capacity?*

10*th* *August 2015*

I don't know what caused me to cry when my TS-clinic check-up at Bath was booked. I know I'm still sensitive about hospitals; all the things that have happened over the past few years. I guess going to the clinic opens those emotional wounds. Sometimes I try and run away from the sadness and discomfort. But I just have to accept what has happened and only hope for the future.

When my appointment came around four days later, the TS team suggested a new medication called Rapamycin, to shrink TS and LAM tumours and cysts. I felt nervous. I didn't want to try a drug that could suppress my immune system and make me more susceptible to infections. If I tried it, I may have to change my epilepsy medication as there could be some side effects. It was too much information to take in and process.

3rd September 2015

I'm holding on tightly to my body. I'm afraid of it. I'm afraid of the unknown, and I'm subconsciously wrapping my arms around my chest protectively. I have to let myself feel the aches and pains. I have to put trust into my body and let go of the need to control it. I have to be ok with the unknown. When I had anxiety before these all these lung operations, I was scared of the unknown then. When I accepted that life is how it is, I relaxed and was able to accept things as they are. I can do that again. I just need to be gentle and patient with myself.

As I looked back at 2015 it was relief that it was over. I had multiple operations, felt sickness and intense pain; but Mencap deferred my start day from September to November and my breathing was improving.

2016

12th May 2016

I was filled with such anxiety this morning. It was a lovely clear spring day, but we were going to Nottingham. I listened to my iPod for comfort and just wanted some quiet while I sat in the back of the car. At the service station I treated myself to a hot chocolate and a magazine. Mum, Dad and I had our sandwiches in the car when we got to the hospital.

I didn't enjoy my lung function test. The skin around my chest wall felt pulled and I had this peg on my nose and a mouthpiece to breathe into. I'm sure this made the lung tests even harder.

I breathed in as much as I could, and then out, I hated the idea of my lungs squeezing out as much air as they could. Oooow!

The clinician tried to be encouraging, but I felt like I was being coached by an Olympic trainer. But I was trying my very best, despite almost crying with pain and effort.

After my lung function, I spoke to Mum and Dad. They tried to reassure me that the LAM team wouldn't do lung function tests if it was to cause any damage. It reassured me a little, but not that much.

Almost an hour later I had my check-up with Professor Johnson. He said my lung function had improved, but since it had only been a year since my previous operation, there was still room for development.

Professor Johnson gave me a leaflet on LAM. It took me back to that poster I saw in Bath. The words *progressive disease, eroding, transplants, little treatment* scared me. It was a reality check that LAM isn't all it's cracked up to be.

During the appointment we talked about the Rapamycin medication. I still didn't want to go on it, but I knew that if I went on it now, while my lung health was stable, then it could slow down the progress of it getting worse in the future.

I had to accept there and then that my body wasn't invincible and that this medication could really help me. I wanted to preserve my health the best I could, so I agreed.

15th May 2016

Mum and I had a walk along the river today. We talked about various things but then we talked about LAM and the prospect of starting Rapamycin. I explained how sad I was about coming to terms with having LAM. I thought my operations had 'fixed' me but there is so much more to that. It's such a horrible and destructive disease.

It was good to walk and let go some of those tears and pain that I'd been holding in.

In mid-October I had my pre-Rapamycin appointment at the LAM centre in Nottingham with the dreaded lung function and blood tests. In my clinic appointment Professor Johnson asked how I'd been getting on and I said my breathing was improving. When I confirmed I did want to take Rapamycin, we discussed how the medicine worked and that I would be starting at 1mg per day. My prescription came through in January.

2017

27th January 2017

I feel so overwhelmed. I began my Rapamycin today. I read the leaflet in the box and scared myself with the possibility of mouth ulcers and all the immune suppressant details – I hate germs anyway, and now I feel more vulnerable to them.

10th February 2017

It's been two weeks since I've been on Rapamycin and my stress levels have been going up and down. Today I had a blood test to see how well I'm responding the drug. It was nice Dad came and gave me some moral support.

March

Just over a month later I had completed my first eight-week box of Rapamycin and I was back at Nottingham for more tests. Sharon, the nurse, came to see how I was getting on. I explained I had a few loose bowel movements and some mouth ulcers, but that things were ok.

After a urine test, I had my check-up with Professor Johnson. We went through the chest x-ray I had back in October and noticed the tiny air pocket on my left lung was gradually getting smaller, since I was doing more exercise. I was really pleased.

30th March 2017

I was a bit worried when Sharon phoned me at work. She reassured me that I was ok, but that the level of Rapamycin in my blood was quite low and asked if I wanted to go up another 1mg. I knew the medicine would be effective if I did, but I still worry about those funny side effects on my immune system.

Sharon and I agreed that I would be upping my dosage the following week and that I would need another blood test two weeks after that.

May

As far as I knew my body was tolerating the Rapamycin well, but by mid-May I was having some funny Focal-impaired seizures, where I remembered the aura of the seizure but not what happened after. My parents got in contact with the hospitals in Bath and Nottingham, who agreed that the Rapamycin was interacting with my epilepsy medication; one of the common side effects I was warned about.

Firstly, my epilepsy medication increased, but that only made my seizures worse. After some trial and error, I changed my epilepsy tablets and after my next appointments in Bath and Nottingham, my MRI scan and chest x-ray results showed that the Rapamycin had begun to shrink the size of the tumours in my brain, and kidneys and lung cysts.

It is a real relief that my health is currently stable. I continue to take Rapamycin and it is still showing positive results. Over the last five years, I've been able to brave the swimming pool again, and have done a lot of walking with the people I support at Mencap. Walking up those gentle hills everyday really helped to develop a lung capacity that I now consider as good-as-normal.

A major achievement for me, was in October 2018 when Mum and I went on one our long walks, and I walked up a 400 ft grassy hill. Being able to look up at the hill from the bottom and challenge it with my stronger lungs and pounding feet, made the achievement of reaching the top a big one.

Meeting Others with LAM

Coming to terms with LAM has been difficult and at times lonely. Back in 2016, just as I was preparing to take Rapamycin, I was feeling quite down and had asked at my previous health-check up in Nottingham, if there was a way of getting in touch with people who have LAM as well.

2016

At the beginning of December, I heard from a woman called Helen, who got in contact with me via email.

> Hi Zoë,
> Jan Johnson from LAM Action has asked me to contact you. I gather you have TSC-LAM and wanted to touch base with another LAM patient who is already on Rapamycin. I have LAM and was diagnosed 8 years ago following numerous chest infections and a pneumothorax. I have been seeing Professor Johnson for most of this time.
>
> I remember only too well how scared I was when was first diagnosed and first started on Rapamycin but believe me it's ok. I would be more than happy to meet up with you if you fancied it?
>
> Drop me a line or give me a call whenever you want to.
>
> All the best,
>
> Helen

6th December 2016

It was really nice to hear from a person who also has LAM.
Helen was really friendly, and I already feel less isolated and
not so worried about taking Rapamycin. She sent me another
email later in the day, asking me if I wanted to go along to a
small gathering at a local garden centre tomorrow, but as it
was short notice, I politely declined, instead saying I would
still like us meet up in the future. She was happy with that.

2019

As I adapted to living with LAM, I felt ready at the start of
the year to get back in touch with Helen and see if we could
meet up.

5th February 2019 (9.51am)

Hi Helen,

I emailed you about two years ago about having LAM.
Sorry it's been a while. I think I have still been coming to
terms with the diagnosis, as well as having TS, and like you
said in your email, it can seem quite scary.

I'm planning to come to the LAM Annual General Meeting
in June. Is that an event you will be attending?

I also feel more ready to meet other people with LAM on a
social level, so if any of your local group will be meeting in
the near future, could you let me know?

Thanks,

Zoë

February 5th 2019 (13.15pm)

Hi Zoë

It is lovely to hear from you. How are you?

Yes, I'm going to the LAM General Meeting in June. I am so glad you are planning on attending. You will get a lot from it I promise.

We haven't got any local meetings yet, but in the meantime if you could like to meet for a coffee, I am more than happy to.

All the best, Helen

After some further emails, Helen and I agreed to meet in *Costa* the following month. In the meantime, I had heard about another local LAM group who meet up in London. I contacted LAM Action, who put me in touch with the woman who ran the regional group.

March

At the start of the year I had no idea that March would involve not only one LAM social meeting, but two. I was pleased with myself for gradually making some connections.

13ᵗʰ March 2019

It was great to finally meet Helen today. We met at the Westgate shopping centre and talked about our experiences with LAM. She was really helpful and inspiring, and I felt supported. A new friendship begins.

23ʳᵈ March 2019

I had been looking around for the café in St Pancras for almost an hour before deciding I might as well go home. I was disappointed because I was beginning to feel excited about this, and if I hadn't walked past a hotel in the station, I wouldn't have noticed the group of ladies I was meeting with.

I felt shy, and I noticed that I was probably one of the youngest people there. They all seemed to be around 15 years older than me, but I guess I'm used to that being the youngest in my family and on my counselling course.

The ladies made me feel welcome and I explained my difficulty in finding the café. They apologised which was nice.

I heard about their stories with LAM; some diagnosed 10 years ago, some recently, others who didn't know they had LAM and now carried cylinders of oxygen with them. I was a bit unsure of how to deal with this all.

When I had my turn, I said I had Tuberous Sclerosis as well. The group had heard about it but none of them had it themselves. I felt disappointed and wondered whether I belonged here. They all had a sporadic version, not the TS-related one.

After spending an hour in the café, I thanked the ladies and agreed to meeting up with them in the future. I knew deep down it would be good for me that I did, even if I was feeling apprehensive at the time.

As I looked out of the window, the racing city scenery merging into long stretches of fields, hills and countryside, I considered how I was still adapting. I was surprised, if not a bit scared to see varying degrees of the condition, and that perhaps because LAM is so rare, that there was even less research was around when these women were growing up. Maybe the disease had progressed further for them than it had for me? I had only heard of LAM because of TS and had some vague awareness that in my early twenties I may have some issues. But for the group I had just met, they could have had LAM for years but not even known.

June

15th June 2019

I went to my first LAM AGM in Watford today. Helen agreed to meet me in the reception and introduced me to some of her friends. I caught up with some familiar faces from the London meeting back in March and it was a great opportunity to meet other young women with LAM too. I thought it was just going to be me, but now it feels more like something we are all experiencing together.

Although reading the research slides about both the sporadic and TS-related versions of LAM was challenging to absorb, I was inspired by how everyone was learning to manage their own version of the condition.

After attending the event, I wrote 1000 words on my experience of the day. I thought about how I had met Jill Pateman, who was the administrator for LAM Action, and that if I emailed this document to her, it could be published in the next issue of LAM Post, the charity's newsletter.

16th June 2019: 15:40pm

This is brilliant Zoë.

I'm really pleased the meeting was a positive experience for you.

I've forwarded your article to the editor of LAM Post. I know he will be very grateful.

Best wishes,

Jill

I was over the moon to get such a prompt and positive response. In the years before, I had been scared and uncertain about LAM, but now I was beginning to celebrate the condition through an article that was published in the 2019 summer issue of LAM Post.

CHAPTER 5

TSC AND MENTAL HEALTH

TSC-Associated Neuropsychiatric Disorders (TAND)

According to the Tuberous Sclerosis Association (TSA), 90% of TSC affected people can develop mental health problems throughout their life. The TSA have categorised this as TSC-Associated Neuropsychiatric Disorders (TAND).

The term may sound overwhelming and scary, but it highlights conditions that many of us are already aware of, whether a person has TSC or not:

– Autistic Spectrum Disorder (ASD)
– Attention Deficient Hyperactivity Disorder (ADHD)
– Anxiety

Just because these conditions are listed, doesn't mean that everyone with TSC will develop them. Some people may do, while others may just experience one or two, if at all.

Autistic Spectrum Disorder

The TSA believe that between 25-50% of the TSC population may develop Autism. While research is still being made about the condition, it is suggested to be more common in Tuberous Sclerosis Complex than it is for the general public. Possible reasons for this may be due to how the brain functions with people who have TSC. Overall, a person with Autism may struggle with changes in their routine, recognising emotions, socialising and stimulating environments.

Attention Deficient Hyperactivity Disorder (ADHD)

As with Autism, ADHD affects more people with TSC than it does to the general population. ADHD may involve a person having an overactive mind, impulsive behaviour and issues following instructions. For example, an ADHD child with TSC may struggle to listen in class or with taking in a lot of information, such as taking on multiple tasks.

Anxiety

It's important to note that anxiety is different to stress. The mental health charity, *Mind* describes stress as:

"Situations or events that put pressure on us or our reaction to being placed under pressure"

(Mind)

Such pressures could be external – pressure from peers at school to fit in, or by critical parents who want their child to perform to perfection; the child never feeling good enough. Or other pressures, which can be internal; the high expectations we can put on ourselves to look perfect or live a life without room for error and acceptance of what we can't change. We can even feel pressured by time, to achieve a task as quickly as possible.

On the other hand:

"Anxiety is what we feel when we are worried or afraid about things that are about to happen or may

*happen in the future. It is a natural human response when
we perceive we are under threat."*

(Mind)

The NHS describes how anyone can become anxious, especially around times of exams or going to a hospital appointment or starting a new job. These occasional bouts of anxiety are common but can become an issue if the symptoms are affecting everyday life activities that might not have bothered you in the past. For example, going out of the house might seem like a challenge when it wasn't before. Or symptoms of a fast heartbeat or muscle tension may be present during the most mundane activities like commuting to and from work or having a cup of tea. If anxiety becomes a problem, usually these symptoms can seem like they come out of the blue for no reason and feel like they are taking over your life.

Common mental health disorders include:

- Generalised Anxiety Disorder (GAD)
- Panic Disorder
- Social Anxiety Disorder
- Obsessive Compulsive Disorder (OCD)
- Health Anxiety
- Post-Traumatic Stress Disorder (PTSD)
- Phobias

For further details about these disorders, information can be accessed via the mental health charity *Mind,* but for the following chapter, I write about my experiences with both Generalised Anxiety Disorder and Health Anxiety.

How is anxiety is connected to TSC?

As with any person who has a long-term condition it is common for health to be at the forefront of the mind. For example, worries around upcoming appointments, medication or fears of becoming unwell. Obsessively thinking about health or regularly checking for symptoms of potential ill health could be early signs of Health Anxiety, whereas Generalised Anxiety Disorder tends to revolve around excessive worries about many areas of a person's life. The TSA indicate that 50% of people with TSC will develop an anxiety disorder in their lifetime.

Cognitive Behavioural Therapy (CBT)

Although there are many available ways to manage anxiety, stress and other mental health issues, such as depression, a common therapy used is called Cognitive Behavioural Therapy.

"CBT is based on the idea that how we think (cognition), how we feel (emotion) and how we act (behaviour) all interact together. Specifically, our thoughts determine our feelings and behaviour"

(Simply Psychology)

CBT was initially a combination of two types of therapy: Rational Emotional Behaviour Therapy (REBT) created by American Psychologist, Albert Ellis in the 1950s, and Cognitive Therapy, designed by American Psychiatrist, Aaron Beck in the 1960s.

REBT was about helping the client view their irrational thoughts and behaviours into more realistic beliefs. For example, a person may think – something dreadful is about to happen if I read a book (thought) so I will avoid reading books (behaviour).

Ellis talks about an ABC model, starting with an activating event that may have caused the irrational belief in the first place:

Activating Event: A person may have had an unexpected seizure while reading a book.

Belief: Every time I read a book; I will have a seizure.

Consequence: Avoidance of reading any book to prevent having seizures.

Although it may seem that the activating event is the issue, Ellis believed that it was the irrational belief that caused the emotional and behavioural responses, such as avoidance of an activity. The understanding was, that if the client became aware of their unhelpful thought, then they could begin to see how realistically simply reading a book didn't mean it was 100% likely a seizure would happen. Over time, the client could gradually start reading again as they gained confidence in their realistic belief.

In terms of Cognitive Therapy, Aaron Beck believed that our thoughts can influence how we see ourselves. If our thoughts are negative "I'm not a good person", then this could cause the patient to believe in that thought and could potentially develop depression. The aim for the therapist was to help their client challenge those negative beliefs through exploration of where those negative thoughts may have come from and how valid they really are.

With the cognitive, emotional and behavioural connections, CBT helps to address those irrational beliefs, either about a potentially threatening event or how a person sees themselves, to a more realistic viewpoint. "I may not be perfect, and that's ok".

From an anxiety perspective, CBT can help challenge those unhelpful avoidance behaviours we can become involved in, such as avoidance of reading a book. Through setting an overall goal and steps to achieve that outcome, the client can gradually expose themselves to the very situation they are afraid of and reduce their fear. The outcome may not be instant, but with patience, it is possible to see an improvement.

This is what I came to explore in my anxiety journey.

My Experiences: Anxiety

I remember sitting at a clinic appointment in Bath and seeing the word *Anxiety* on a leaflet. The description of it sounded like stress x 1000.

2009

I had begun sixth form college in the September of 2009. It was great to have my secondary school friends come with me and also make new friends in my Creative and Media class. I was bit nervous though, making a new start in preparation for university in two years' time.

By December, we knew this would be the last Christmas that Granny would be alive. She was becoming more and more frail and had recently had a heart attack.

2010

After the turn of the new decade in 2010, I was becoming more and more worried about Granny's health and whether we would lose her before we thought we would. After she had been checked over in the hospital, she was diagnosed with Ovarian Cancer and all this fragility began to make more sense. Prior to this, I had never needed to prepare myself for losing a relative, but it caused more anxiety than I would have ever imagined.

One January evening, not long after the news I began hyperventilating. The air was stuffy, and my heart was beating, at what felt like a million miles per hour; the sound of blood pounding in my ears. Hot tears were pouring down my cheeks in panic as I sat on the edge of my parents' bed as they encouraged me to calm down. *"Take deep breaths out"*, Mum was saying. I was scared that I would be having a heart attack aged sixteen.

I continued breathing deeply with Mum, while Dad offered to take my blood pressure with his blood pressure monitor. *"It's just a little high, but nothing to worry about."* Dad confirmed. Hearing that helped me to calm down more and my breathing began slowing down and returning to normal. I felt exhausted.

On the 1st April, Granny had made it to her 90th birthday. We had a family celebration and by then I had begun to adjust to the possibility that each time I saw her could be the last. A few days later my parents and I went to Disney World for two weeks. We had a great time until we heard that a volcano in Iceland was spitting out a black ash cloud that was preventing us getting our flight back home.

We checked out of our Disney hotel and booked into a smaller one outside of the Disney park for couple of days to see how we could get home. Dad bought a cheap laptop and found us a cruise ship that was sailing across the Atlantic. He hired a car to drive five hours down to Fort Lauderdale at the southern point of the Florida coast. It was a whirlwind of a time and I just wanted to get home.

On the morning of 20th April, I was reflecting over a vivid dream I had had the previous night. The scene was black and there was a white glow coming from a door on the right. Granny with her cloud of white curled hair was dressed in her grey coat, with a long dark skirt peeping from underneath, black shoes and her classic red lipstick on. She had a brown suitcase with her. She hugged me and told me that she was going....

My parents called me from the bathroom because they had some news. *"I know...she's died. I had a dream about her last night."* I called through the door as I stepped out of the bathroom. A spiritual experience or simply a coincidence? It was a special moment that even in my mind, Granny was taking the time to let me know she was ready to die, and, in a way, I was allowing her to.

The crossing over the Atlantic was therapeutic, blue sky and blue sea for six days. Although that time allowed for deep reflection, I felt emotionally numb, still unable to cry. The funeral arrangements were taking place back in England for when we returned. I sang Faith Hill's song *There You'll Be,* accompanied by Geoffrey on his guitar, at the service. At the end of the day I was truly able to let myself cry out my deep feelings towards my Granny's death.

Struggling with Anxiety

The following months were smoother. The weather was getting warmer and I was able to enjoy college and assist a local photographer at some weddings for work-experience over the holidays.

Before college started again in the autumn term, my parents and I took a late summer break to the Lake District in early September. We stayed for a week in small town near Lake Windermere in a little apartment. The building was quite dated and had a musky smell and furniture that reminded me of Granny. I thought I was over her death by now.

Despite walks along beautiful streams, wooded landscapes and attractions like Beatrix Potter's house, I felt a growing knot of tension in my diaphragm. Wasn't my body supposed to be relaxed in this blissful environment? I tried listening to my favourite music in the car, but the tension grew tighter and tighter the more I tried to escape it. I began to worry that this tension would affect my health and I began worrying about the possibility of hyperventilating again like I did at the beginning of the year. This was the beginning of a vicious cycle of how I dealt with anxiety.

2011

After keeping a journal for one year and noticing I was running out of room to write about my anxieties on just one page, I decided to buy an additional notebook to be my stress journal. This would be an unlimited space for me to write at length about how I have been feeling and come to terms about where my anxiety is coming from.

9th January 2011

...I've heard stress is wasted energy. Why am I wasting it on worrying about being stressed? Sometimes when I'm so stressed, I worry about January last year and hyperventilating and heart attacks. Surely worrying about my health isn't doing it any good. What if it leads to heart disease later in life? What if I have a heart attack? I know if I can allow myself to relax I will.

I'm trying to control it though. I went to my doctor last week who took my blood pressure officially. He said I was fine and that has reassured me. Sometimes I can watch a film for an hour and then, when I realise I've been relaxed I tense up again. It's like I want to be in control, but I know if I let my body do its own thing, I will be fine. I shouldn't have to worry. I need to trust myself...

Over the following months, my anxiety and thoughts were like a rollercoaster up and down; some days relaxed, some days tense and panicky. I began searching for positive quotes to uplift and inspire me on my bad days, ones about not letting anxiety get me down and that I'm strong enough to overcome this. I was worried that reading about my anxiety would set it off with more tension and worried thoughts. I wanted to avoid anxiety has much as possible.

At the end of July, Sarah had got married and for at least this month I had felt calmer. The event provided enough excitement and distraction from my anxious thoughts and tension, but that didn't last for long on the approach to starting my first year at university.

The transition from further to higher education seemed scary. My friendship groups would be dispersing all over the country and there would be so many different faces to get to know in a new place of study. Fortunately, everyone was kind and supportive of each other on the photography course and I was feeling happier. I felt comforted that I could just catch a train to and from London each day as I wasn't ready to live in student accommodation.

2012

At the beginning of the year stressful course deadlines and lack of sleep began to affect my anxiety levels again. My diaphragm was growing tense and I was overthinking my breathing pattern, unable to focus on anything else. It was around this time that I began learning about mindfulness and how the worries we often have relate to what we have done in the past or what we are concerned about in the future. I was certainly worried something awful may happen to me in the future which I was trying to prevent through worrying. By using mindfulness, I learnt that knitting is a great way to promote relaxation in the present moment while doing an activity. I bought some wool and Mum taught me the basic garter stitch. Although I didn't have a project in mind, simply wrapping the wool around the needles helped reduce my stress levels.

At times I still found myself avoiding the possibility of my anxiety returning, but that only seemed to promote it more. I gained some clarity when the summer came. I created a motivation board with all the positive quotes that I had been collecting so it could spur me on while I tried living at university in my second year.

2013

By January I had been staying in university accommodation for several months, but anxiety was still bothering me. I would sit on the bus to the university campus, the tension across my diaphragm tightening like a belt. Once again I tried to distract it with relaxing music, but *the belt* got tighter and tighter the more I struggled out of it. I wrote in my stress journal before I moved back to London after Christmas:

4th January 2013

What am I worried about? I'm worried I'm going to be stressed forever. The ECG I had said I was fine. I need to calm down and not feel rushed trying to relax as soon as possible...

By February my nervous system was still up and down - good days, bad days and everything in between.

10th February 2013

I'm starting to find patterns. I'm forcing myself to relax. I'm trying to be perfect and stress-free the whole time but it's just not happening. No one's body is relaxed all the time, but I just want to be calm. Frustration is half of it, the tension just won't disappear because I ask it to.

16th February 2013

I feel sluggish. I feel like a person in their old age, not someone is going to be twenty in April. Maybe I'm just so tensed up that I'm not getting enough oxygen around my body? I'm

RARE: A JOURNEY OF SELF-ACCEPTANCE

feeling thin like I'm not getting enough nutrients. Even my jeans are becoming baggy.

25 February 2013

After a week of misery and anxiety I can feel a wave of a better feelings. I saw a shop called "Fresh Start". Looking at that sign I feel happier and healthier and it motivated me to go to the gym. After that twenty minutes I noticed that my cheeks felt pink and my body didn't seem so numb anymore. I feel like a nineteen-year-old again.

4th March 2013

I woke up today and I felt relaxed. As soon as I thought that, I could feel the tension and panic returning, its grip getting tighter and tighter again. My relaxed state was disappearing. But instead of sliding completely into the scary abyss of sluggish torture, I remembered reading about self-care and that by treating myself well, I could help reduce my anxiety. I made myself a good breakfast with some fresh orange juice and Weetabix, drizzled with honey and blueberries. I made my bed and folded my blanket up like it would be in a hotel.

I found a sense of control that boosted my confidence; I began to make time for meditation and yoga in my student flat; I was knitting a patchwork blanket for my expected nephew due in May. I discovered that if I ate healthy foods and reduced sugar and fat in my diet, I would be keeping my heart healthy from all the stress I have been giving it, but I was continuing to lose weight.

General Anxiety Disorder (GAD) Diagnosis/ Cognitive Behavioural Therapy (CBT)

I thought that being in control meant that it would *cure* my anxiety, but in April, during the Easter Holidays, Mum and I went to the doctor's to discuss my high stress levels and my inability to relax. Dr Keast made a referral for Cognitive Behavioural Therapy (CBT) that resolves negative thinking patterns into a positive mindset.

I felt embarrassed about going to therapy. It felt like a weakness, admitting that I needed help. None of my friends had therapy; they were all fine. Deep down I knew that I had tried my hardest to cope with my feelings without professional help and surrendering to a therapist seemed like the next available option. I waited until June when my referral came through and began my first of six sessions of CBT at the end of the month.

Session 1

When I arrived at *Talking Therapies*, I received a warm smile from the receptionist. While I waited, I filled in an anxiety and depression form noting down how I had been feeling over the past two weeks, and it was given to my therapist.

She called my name and I went into her room. I was nervous but ready to talk. We went through a contract, promising that our work would be private and confidential. I was then given the opportunity to talk about how I had been feeling over the past few years: Granny's death, hyperventilating, trying to cope with anxious thoughts and a tense diaphragm. I couldn't believe I was sharing such personal information with a person I had just met - I had only told my parents about it all in January.

My therapist was kind and asked me what I wanted to get out of our sessions. I explained how I didn't want to be worried anymore. I expected my worries about anxiety and heart attacks to be judged as nonsense, but I appreciated that she acknowledged my irrational perceptions with all seriousness.

We discussed my results on the anxiety and depression form. I had scored 13 out of 27 for mild depression and 16 out of 21 for anxiety, which was in the severe range. Lisa* informed me that I have General Anxiety Disorder (GAD).

I was disappointed to discover I had an anxiety disorder, but it made complete sense; I worried all the time and it *was* getting the way of my day-to-day life. I was given a guided relaxation CD and handed a CBT Workbook. The book illustrated situations that influence the thoughts we have; the physical and emotional reactions that take place which impact the behaviours.

Setting Therapeutic Goals

Apart from the first planning session, the other sessions would take place once a week over the phone and I would fill in the CBT workbook for my homework. By reading through the book I discovered that setting goals could be a helpful way of improving my wellbeing. My first idea was to write a list of my achievements over my therapeutic journey.

Achievements

19/4/13 – Went to the doctor's to request some therapy.

12/6/13 – Spoke to Talking Therapies on the phone about my first therapy session.

20/6/13 – 1st session at Talking Therapies.

25/6/13 – Set 1st SMART goal. Emailed wedding photographer about work-experience.

28/6/13 – 1st week of therapy complete.

4/7/13 – Felt relaxed and was able to breathe.

Health Anxiety

I was able to relax during a holiday in France with my parents and our family friends, the Daveys. I enjoyed taking photos of

Notre-Dame on my black and white film camera and eating at fancy restaurants in the evening. It was being on holiday that gave me the realisation that my worries have been health related. Granny's illness and death was an initial trigger, but then I began to worry about the negative impact stress could have on my own health. I'd always hated health check-ups and my epilepsy scared me.

As my CBT workbook suggested, I realised I that my efforts of *controlling* my anxiety were actually avoidance techniques. I had been pounding the treadmill at the gym to run away from the emotional and physical discomfort of my anxiety. I was eating a predominantly green diet to avoid feeling the unhealthy effects of my prolonged stress. With all this avoidance, I was just fuelling my nervous system with more stress, creating a vicious cycle.

A few days after I got home from my holiday, I had my second therapy phone session. I explained my revelation that I want to deal with my health anxieties.

17th July 2013

My therapist emailed me a link to a Health Anxiety workbook with modules about how to deal with it. What a relief she had some resources up her sleeve.

The workbook was just what I needed. It had nine modules and on the same day, I had already read what Health Anxiety was and how it develops. I wrote about my reflections:

"Experiences that have increased my health anxiety are having TS and seizures from a young age. I have always had hospital visits and medication. Granny dying of cancer heightened my anxiety as I had never experienced a death in the family before."

I discovered that I had created unhelpful beliefs about my health, that I believed a mild sensation in my chest or increased heart rate meant I would have a heart attack, and that my response in tensing up was way of protecting myself. I had become afraid of that tension and my response to that would be to worry about the initial trigger – a perceived heart attack.

I wrote down my list of avoidance tactics around my obsessive green eating and exercising habits. I explored my safety behaviours of wrapping my arm over my stomach while holding on to my jumper, biting down on my tongue or controlling my breathing pattern. I thought these things would take my mind off constantly focusing on my body, but the workbook informed me that avoidance only provides short-term relief. I wanted long-term relief.

My belief was that the more I focused on my body, the more I could catch out health warnings, but I was focusing on the wrong part of my health. My heart health was fine, but my right kidney wasn't. Simply focusing on my anxiety symptoms didn't protect me as I still became unwell when my kidney bled.

My anxiety levels had been gradually coming back down but after my embolisation, I was hyper-aware of my back and whether any inkling of pain was my kidney; I was also iron deficient, so I felt pale and lethargic. It was times like these when focusing on my health was a good thing and I could address all my worries at the same time.

<u>24th September 2013</u>

CBT Thought Diary:
What am I worried about? – I'm worried about my kidney.
What am I predicting? - That it will happen again.
What emotions am I feeling? – Fear, uncertainty, anxiety.

What action will take if the worst happens: Seek medical attention immediately.

Challenging unhelpful thoughts:

Factual evidence for thought: The event has already happened.

Factual evidence against thought: As it has happened it may not happen again.

Explanation of symptoms: I have been ill recently, and my body is probably still adjusting as I recover.

As well as filling in diagrams and thought diaries, I also began to address my reassurance checking behaviours and tried to reduce them.

<u>27th September 2013</u>

<u>What are my reassurance and safety behaviours?</u>
- *Checking for palpations*
- *Muscle tension*
- *Checking blood pressure*
- *Researching symptoms online*

<u>Negative Consequences to checking:</u>
- *Too much checking will cause more anxiety*
- *My muscles will get tighter*
- *I can't always rely on articles to be scientifically correct*

Over the next month I focused my attention on my mindful hobbies including yoga, knitting and illustrating my anxiety symptoms through photography for my degree. I also began some exposure practice in which I picked one of my fears and worked through it step by step. As blood pressure was a key worry, I worked on that first.

Towards the end of my therapy I began expanding my focus onto other areas of my life with a *healthy living* worksheet, as part of my workbook.

In my discharge letter I was able to see in scientific terms how my anxiety and depression levels had fluctuated between June and October 2013. I began in the severe range of General Anxiety Disorder with a score of 16; a moderate range score of 14 the following week, before dropping to mild score of 11 the week after. I could really see my progress.

After the first three therapy sessions both my GAD and depression scores continued to decrease, peaking slightly in August after my kidney operation. By late September my scores were in the normal mental health range, but I continued to fill in my workbook for another month.

25th October 2013

I've just completed my sixth therapy session. It felt like it was time to go my own way and my therapist was really impressed with how well I have coped, particularly through my operation recovery. The great thing was that she told me that I had done the work myself and that she had just been there to listen.

It's amazing how I've turned this around. I remember phoning the doctor's in June and I felt very lost and scared that life was whipping up a frenzy that was destroying me.

Things started to turn around after coming out of hospital and how my therapist told me about a man who was too afraid to do his shopping because walking through the carpark gave him panic attacks. By exposing himself to his fears he became more confident about walking through the carpark. He was empowering himself, not giving that power away to his fear.

I learnt from my therapy that it is about facing anxious feelings head on and being able to sit with the discomfort without viewing it as a threat. It's choosing not to react, rather than ignoring it.

I'm a little scared about this freedom, but I'm bound to be. If I feel tense, I'm just going to acknowledge it and let it be. I can do this. I have done this!

It's easy to imagine that going through a workbook and having therapy sessions would fix everything once and for all. The truth is, I still get anxious from time to time. Sometimes that belt of tension is non-existent, sometimes it is gently resting around my diaphragm, and occasionally it feels really tight. But that is no fault of my own or of Cognitive Behavioural Therapy. The reality is, there is no cure, but rather what I have learned through my therapeutic journey, is that I have gathered tools to help me manage and deal with anxious feelings when they are arise.

As I highlighted in my October journal entry, allowing yourself to feel your all emotions, rather than avoiding or resisting them, gives you more power. It is acceptance.

> *"It's not what happens to you, but how you react to it that matters"*
>
> *Epictetus*

CHAPTER 6

EDUCATION

TSC & Special Educational Needs (SENs)

Entering education can be a big step for any child. With conditions such as Tuberous Sclerosis Complex (TSC), this step can seem even greater. As everyone with TSC is affected differently, some children may not have any learning issues, while others may need regular support.

Learning difficulties and learning disabilities might be an issue when it comes to education for a TSC-affected child, however these may present themselves in various ways. There may be a certain area of learning that a child finds challenging such as reading, writing or counting numbers. For others managing emotions or speech development may be difficult, whilst hearing or visual deficiencies might be a concern in the classroom. The Tuberous Sclerosis Association (TSA) has highlighted these areas as Special Educational Needs (SENs) and provides information care plans that help to support people in the different stages of their education.

Although care plans may not be needed for every TSC-affected child, some children may just need support in the classroom by a teaching assistant or keyworker, while others can work independently. Whether a child attends mainstream, or a specialised school will depend on the individual.

Further details about learning disabilities and learning difficulties are included in a chapter on Mencap.

My Experiences

Early Years and Primary School

Despite having seizures as an infant, my intellectual ability was in the range of the general population. I had the standard "two-year test" to see if my progress was in line with other infants my age, but had a few struggles with stacking bricks and jigsaw puzzles, but over time I gradually found these tasks easier.

In the years before I started school, I went to a local childminder and developed my independence and creative side with arts and crafts. I took those skills on to pre-school and then primary school and settled in well.

With the creative side of school coming easy to me, I loved English and writing stories, however I didn't enjoy Maths and Science very much. Numbers weren't my friends, but I was too shy to ask for help.

"Zoë is very quiet in class, but outside she has a really loud playground voice. It would great if we encouraged that playground voice to make some contribution in class." – That was often what my teachers would say at parents' evenings, and I would feel even more embarrassed hearing that back. I couldn't help being shy, but I listened well in class and received a "Good Listener" certificate from my teacher. At least my quiet nature was being recognised as something good.

In order to develop my Maths skills, I had a tutor, before trying out a Japanese tutoring system, *Kumon*. For a few years, towards the end of primary school and the first years of secondary school, I worked on a short *Kumon* maths paper every day after breakfast.

The addition, subtraction and multiplication sums were easy in a horizontal form but when they became stacked on top of each other and various digits had to be crossed out to get the answer, it was more complicated. *Kumon* helped me feel more confident at those sums, as well as fractions and percentages. But long division sums still weren't my favourite.

Completing a paper everyday was annoying but having to go to the community centre every week for a longer paper was even more frustrating. I hated the teacher, simply for being associated with Maths, and I hated having to do more Maths than everyone else did in my class.

Secondary School

At secondary school, I was reacquainted with my friend, Helen, who has Cerebral Palsy. Helen was two months older than me and our families had met in hospital when we were young, sharing a takeaway pizza.

While a lot of my peers were a bit nervous around Helen with her unsteady gait and tucked-in-arm, those elements didn't bother me, and I often stood up for her when she got bullied. For the next five years in our tutor group, we sat next to each other and talked about our shared love for horse riding and became great friends.

Helen and I weren't in many classes together though, so I was a bit lonely before I truly felt welcomed into a friendship group. But while Helen was in the class below me for Maths, English and Science, my other friends were in the groups above me. So, I was somewhere floating in the middle.

Although asking for help was something I continued to struggle with throughout school, I passed most of my subjects at GCSE level. I felt pleased for getting full marks in my

Geography exam, and that I could say more in French than just:

"Bonjour, je m'appelle Zoë. Parlez-vous anglais?"

With my big hopes of me achieving an A in Art, my teacher went on maternity leave and I missed her encouraging, yet constructive feedback on my coursework. Although I passed with a C, and I don't even remember what project I made for my final art GCSE piece, the best achievement for me was in Year 10 when my 1x1 metre mixed-media-collage of London was unexpectedly chosen to be put onto the wall in my headteacher's office. It felt like a really proud moment, and I enjoyed peeking through the side window of his office when I walked into school each morning

English Language and English Literature were my best subjects where I got two Bs. Science, I did well, and I.T, but I still missed out on a C for Maths. *Was I ever going to get it?*

College

In sixth-form college I had the opportunity to re-take my Maths GCSE and after a year, finally passed with a C. Being in the middle Maths class at school, our ability varied quite a bit, so in retrospect, I probably could have got the grade first time if had been brave enough to ask for help. But as my GCSE Maths college class was full of people of a similar ability and struggled with similar equations, I was less embarrassed about asking for help because I didn't feel I came across so bad for not understanding it first time round. It was just a relief to finally get that subject out of the way of my education.

While I was re-taking my Maths GCSE, instead of A-Levels I took a Level 3 diploma in Creative Media. It was a fantastic two-year course where I could explore a whole range of creative subjects, from photography to graphic design and animation.

I knew from the day after I left secondary school that I wanted to be a wedding photographer. My cousin, Mark, was getting married and I was blown away by his wife's fairy-tale wedding dress and bridesmaid dresses; the beautiful hotel and gardens; the wedding cake. *Wouldn't that be amazing as a job?*

University

In the summer months at college, I took on work experience with a local photographer. It was a great opportunity see how a real wedding photographer worked and I couldn't wait to get started myself. I was elated when Sarah and her fiancé, Phil, said I could take their official engagement photos and family friends allowed me to take unofficial pictures at their weddings as well.

When I got to university, I had a reality check about photography. As much I enjoyed being an assistant at a Hindu wedding photography company and experimenting with 35mm film in the darkroom, I was ignoring some of the basic details of a photography career. My parents had bought me whole set of professional studio photography equipment; the spotlights, the white backdrop-everything. I was grateful, if not overwhelmed, but I was beginning to doubt myself. Did I really want to spend my career setting up lights in studio? It was the technical aspect that I struggled with the most when it came to photography. I couldn't help feeling embarrassed and guilty.

I thought back to one of my first days at university. The head lecturer mentioned how taking photos is only 10% of running a photography business; there is setting up and advertising the company; attaining clients; travelling from venue to venue; editing the photos...

I didn't like telling wedding guests or families - who I didn't know personally - how to stand for their portraits. I felt bossy if I did, and the whole situation seemed so staged and false. I didn't want to run a photography business after all.

2014

In the last months of my degree, I began to realise how much of my photography coursework, images, and essays were psychology related. The photos I took illustrated my experience with anxiety; a portraits project on the identity of people varying in age, gender, sexuality and culture, describing on a A3 whiteboard what their identity meant to them; and my final exhibition project was going to be on the transition of childhood to adulthood – ballet shoes next to a pair of high heels; a toy clock next to an alarm clock.

I thought about when first looked at Mum's book on the zodiac star signs, how fascinated I was by different personalities; I liked the Myers-Briggs personality type system too. Reading about introversion and extraversion when I was sixteen helped me understand the difference between shyness, a mild social anxiety; the need to be alone to recharge (introversion) compared to feeling energised by people (extraversion). I liked photography, but I was more fascinated by the mind.

Within the month after my twenty-first birthday, guilt was still eating away at me. So much money had gone into my degree, my parents had got me all that photography equipment. *They are going to be so cross at me for not wanting to be a photographer anymore.*

Before I spoke to them, I wrote a letter in my journal.

27th April 2014

I've been meaning to talk to you both about what I want to do when I leave uni. On Thursday when I was around at Betty's she asked me what I wanted to do. I told her I wasn't sure but that I was torn between two things: photography and becoming a counsellor.

I said to her that I don't think being a businesswoman is for me and I'd rather do photography as a casual thing. I think I've just been denying my apparent passion for psychology and helping people. I think would suit me a lot more as a day-to-day job.

I know it may mean more studying, but if I look for a job then save up, I could pay for a course myself. I've felt quite guilty about this because we didn't set up the photography studio too long ago and it was a lot of money. I don't want you to think I'm taking it for granted. I still enjoy photography, but don't have the commitment for the business side of it. Just so you know.

I was surprised how understanding my parents were. There was some disappointment in their response, but the overall message was that they have always encouraged Geoffrey, Sarah and I to pursue what we wanted.

I felt really grateful that they understood, and I learnt that before they became teachers, my parents worked in hotel and hospitality, before deciding it wasn't for them. *So they do know what it feels like.*

Graduation

I have always loved in films how when students graduate, they dress up in their robes and throw their mortar boards in the air. I was expecting that's what it would be like, but it wasn't. Many of my peers on my degree turned up but none of my friends. I wanted to share this exciting moment with them, but some were graduating later in the year and others just didn't bother.

Although it wasn't anything personal towards me, it was disappointing that we had all worked hard together and had a good laugh, but this was what we were working for – this graduating moment.

Luckily Mum and Dad came to the conference hall in Wembley Stadium to watch me graduate. I wore a blue and white polka dot sun dress, my black robe and mortarboard, and had my photo taken holding my certificate. Even if my uni friends weren't there, it was a proud moment for me – a person with TS achieving a Bachelor's Degree with Honours in Photography. In a way, I felt like I was achieving it for the TS community and that it is possible to achieve a degree, when at first, I struggled with Maths and asking for help.

On the way home, my parents took me to one of our favourite pubs for dinner and we celebrated with a glass of champagne. It was a mixed celebration because on the one hand I was recognising my achievements, but also, I look back on that day as the last time I could drink alcohol before I went back onto medication.

CHAPTER 7

MENCAP

What is the Royal Mencap Society?

In 1946 'The National Association of Parents of Backward Children' was established by Judy Fryd who had a child with learning disabilities. Fryd set up the charity to reach out to other parents, describing in an article she wrote about how there weren't many services around to support children like her own.

In the 1950s, the association renamed itself, becoming 'The National Society for Mentally Handicapped Children' and a selection of them tried out the experience of living in accommodation that was set out like a home and educational nursery. The outcome of the trial was successful as results showed improvements in mental and social abilities. Further opportunities for children with learning disabilities became available in the creative arts and sports in the late 60s, when 'The National Society for Mentally Handicapped Children' became the Royal Mencap Society, widely known as Mencap.

Over the following decades and into the 21st century, people of all ages with learning disabilities were given equal rights and new employment opportunities, as well as being able to get involved with the Paralympics.

What is a learning disability? – Connections to TSC

Mencap describes a learning disability as:

"A reduced intellectual ability and difficulty in everyday tasks, for example household tasks, socialising or managing money. People with a learning disability tend to take longer to learn and may need support to develop new skills, understand complicated information and interact with other people."

(Mencap 2020)

Mencap point out that a learning disability differs from a learning *difficulty* as a person's intelligence is not affected, but it is common for people to have both a learning disability and learning difficulty. Conditions such as Dyspraxia, and Attention Deficit Hyperactivity Disorder (ADHD) tend to come under the learning *difficulty* category, whereas Dyslexia and issues around understanding language and social cues are classed as a learning disability.

The severity of a learning disability can vary, from:

profound (a person with an IQ below 20)
severe (an IQ between 20-34)
moderate (IQ range 35-49)
mild (an IQ between 50-70)

The Tuberous Sclerosis Association (TSA) suggests that 30% of people with TSC have profound learning disabilities, 20% are in the moderate to mild ranges and the remaining 50% have the same intellectual ability as the general population.

Mencap is one of many charities that the TSA collaborates with regarding learning disabilities. Further information is available on the TSA website.

Supported Living

To help adults with learning disabilities develop their independence, many people go down the route of Supported Living. For more than twenty years, Mencap have been working with their co-charity *Golden Lane Housing,* which runs many of the homes. Both charities describe their approach as treating their clients as individuals and prioritising their safety. Each client is assessed regarding their physical and mental abilities, as well as being supported in where they may want to live and who they may want to live with.

Supported living provides an opportunity for clients to run a normal home life with the added social care when they need it.

Social Care – Care Worker vs. Support Worker

Charities such as Mencap employ Support Workers to help look after their clients. The roles of a Care Worker and Support Worker are often used interchangeably; they are both caring roles and may both help with personal care, such as showering, preparing meals and accessing the community.

However, the main difference between a Care Worker and Support Worker, is that the one role is often found working with the elderly and the physically disabled, whereas the other works with learning disabilities and empowers their clients to lead independent lives.

A Care Worker may be looking after a person who is unable or limited in doing everyday tasks for themselves. They may need help to get out of bed using a hoist or need feeding during mealtimes.

On the other hand, a Support Worker may support a person who needs 24-hour care, or someone who just needs a few hours of support a week. A Support Worker may observe the person they are supporting as they prepare a sandwich, for example. The Support Worker encourages the client to develop their independence but supports them with tasks they may find challenging. These tasks will vary depending on the individual. While one person in Supported Living might be able to make their sandwich themselves, their housemate may need their Support Worker to hold their walking frame steadily, so they can stand up safely and make their own way to the kitchen.

If the Support Worker made a sandwich without asking what their person wanted, and just gave it to them, this could de-skill this person who may be able to make basic decisions for themselves and are physically able to access the kitchen with minimal support.

This is why it is important to consider the individual needs of each person as a Support Worker and record these abilities and limitations down in a personalised Support Plan.

My Experiences

How I became involved with Mencap

2014

It was great to finally have a degree, even if I wasn't going to be a professional Photographer. The summer was long and sunny, and I was beginning to look for jobs in September. Towards the end of the month my left lung collapsed unexpectedly, forcing me spending remainder of the year in and out of hospital recovering from multiple operations.

2015

This year I was coming to terms with being diagnosed with TS-related LAM and as the spring came around, I was gaining physical and emotional energy to start looking for those job opportunities again. I tried shops, small businesses, cafés; strange job titles I wasn't really interested in like a receptionist role at a solicitors, when I knew nothing about law.

In early March, I was finally given an interview for a café that primarily sold cakes and pastries. I was offered a trial shift and I took it.

11th March 2015

My trial shift was awful. I thought I did a good job waiting the tables, but I don't think tears pricking in the back of my eyes is a way to feel about a potential job. One of the waiters tutted at me when I couldn't understand his accent and how I was supposed to learn the floor plan of the tables when I was only working there for an hour?

12th March 2015

I have been feeling down about yesterday. My body is achy, and my throat is sore after several adrenaline-filled days. Part of me blames myself for not getting the job right. I tried my best but I will have to find something better.

The following day, I stumbled across a career skills quiz on the National Careers Service website to find out what area of work was I most suited to. After filling in the questionnaire I discovered I scored highest in the *Working Well with Others* section and my highest interest group was *Caring.*

After considering the possibility of training to become a counsellor the year before, it was amazing to see how my quiz results showed I was interested in working in social care and counselling. It was giving me the confidence to focus on potential jobs I may actually want to do, and Mum mentioned that her friend had noticed a Support Worker role with Mencap in the local newspaper.

19th March 2015

I spent this afternoon working on an application for the Support Worker role. If I get the job, I would be able to get there by train so it could be ideal.

25th March 2015

Good news! I got offered an interview with Mencap this Friday. I'm quite worried though, because I have been offered so many interviews but then not got the job, so my excitement is being held back a bit. It's hard. You get so close to the job, so close to the potential income and then that can be taken away by a phone call to say it wasn't you. Rejection hurts. Someone has got to give me job, somebody does. Will it be Mencap?

I was pleased the interview went well. I was asked lots of questions and got a positive response when I mentioned how supportive I was of Helen's disability throughout school. I just had to hope I would get the job.

Delayed Start Date

April

A few days later my right lung collapsed, and I was in hospital for a week. When I got home, I had an email from Mencap inviting me to my second interview. Despite feeling weak my parents and I composed an email to the Service Manager to update her on the situation.

Thank you for inviting me to a second interview tomorrow.
Yesterday I was discharged from hospital after another lung collapse due to my health conditions. The doctors have said my lung has healed but I need to take it easy for a couple of weeks. I may have a small operation in the near future to prevent it from happening again.

Is it possible I could defer my interview to a later date?

I'm really interested in working with Mencap, particularly having been in hospital recently. Paying attention to how the nurses work with the patients has inspired me even more to help others develop their independence.

I personally feel this will be the best area of work for me where my strengths are my strongest and where it can be most beneficial for others and myself.

I look forward to hearing from you soon,

Zoë

An hour after I had sent my email, the Service Manager responded sending her sympathy and agreeing to defer my second interview. On 24th April, I was offered the job!

Four days later I was back at Guy's Hospital to have my planned operation to secure my right lung. While I was recovering, I received an email from Mencap with my offer letter. Although I felt drained and drowsy from my operation, there was small glow of happiness inside me that my employment was finally official.

June

It was disappointing that I had spent most of May in hospital, but I was glad I could finally come home. Dad suggested that we contact Mencap to update them on my progress and defer my start date.

I'm starting to recover well, and I know we spoke about me starting in July. My doctor suggested that I take July and August to recuperate as I was in hospital longer than expected. Fortunately, my operation was a success and shouldn't cause any more problems. I hope this ok and that my position is still available?

I think my training was going to be this month. Do you know when the next induction training is going to be?

Kind regards,

Zoë

When Linda* got back to me, she said that she had spoken to HR and they had put my application on hold, but it wouldn't affect my employment. *What a relief!*

Considering I had that horrible trial shift at that café back in March, the situation now couldn't have been more different. I felt supported and respected; that my ill health was being taken seriously and Mencap were being patient enough to wait for me to fully recover before they were happy for me to start work.

September

I had spent the summer building my strength and increasing my lung capacity through singing and walking. I emailed Linda to let her know that I was able to resume my application.

Starting at Mencap

November

Throughout October I gone through the admin processes of DBS checks and within the first few days of the month I was beginning my induction training and meeting the people I would be supporting.

2nd November 2015

I went to one of the supportive living homes at Mencap today. My nerves were all jangly on the train there and I just wanted it to go well. I was worried if the people would like me and if they were expecting a more experienced person to be supporting them. They don't know about my health conditions so I know I could just be a 'normal' person to them, but in a way, I kind of felt like an imposter.

I knocked on the door and a child-like-middle-aged-woman let me in and gave me a warm smile. She was one of the people I might be supporting. There were about five other Mencap residents and one of the support workers introduced me to them. They all told me their names and all had such lovely characters. I think I could enjoy working here.

Before I began working with any of the residents officially, I went on a training week in Oxford:

Day 1: Welcome to the Royal Mencap Society

Day 2: Supporting and Safeguarding People
Day 3: Emergency First Aid at Work
Day 4: Medication Administration
Day 5: Fire Theory
Day 6: Manual Handling (people)
Day 7: Knowledge Assessment Day

Looking at the training schedule I felt overwhelmed and nervous meeting other trainees, smiling awkwardly at them. How was I going to learn all this information?

<u>*5ᵗʰ November 2015*</u>

Yesterday we did first aid training and today we did medication administrating. Both days had difficult moments as there was information on choking and seizures. I was reminded of that horrible November evening, four years ago when I had Bronchitis, and then negative memories of seizures from the past. The trainers even mentioned the name of the medication I'm on. That was weird.

Although it was hard, I stuck with it. I know it will make me more aware of how to work with individuals who may be choking or having a seizure. Still scary though.

When going through a pair exercise on administrating medication, we did a role play. I followed the safety procedures but forgot to interact with the 'client'. She pointed this out and explained the best way to go about it is to include the person in the process, saying things like, what your name is and "Are you ready to have your medication now?"

Initially, I saw her comments as a criticism but as she was talking to me, I could see she was just being helpful.

I was relieved when I passed my Knowledge Assessment and I could begin shadowing other Support Workers to get an idea of putting my new skills into practice.

First Shifts

The next week I began my first shadowing shifts. Like on the day I met some of the people I would be supporting, my jangly nerves were returning, and I was filled with beginner's anxiety that I just wanted to run away from.

I got off my train and walked ten minutes to the supported living home where I was going to be doing my first shadowing shift. It was almost nine o clock. The Support Worker from the previous night shift greeted me. She suggested I read the Support Plan of the person I was supporting while I waited for the member of staff I was shadowing to arrive.

Reading every person's Support Plan was an important part of my training. I was learning about who the people were, what their condition(s) were; how they were affected, such as any behavioural problems they had; the medication they took and any specific dietary requirements that had to be followed.

The lady was I supporting on this shift was called Becca*, and I read about how she regularly attended a day centre several days week and how she had a personal day to do her food shopping and tidying around the house. When the Support Worker arrived, he introduced himself as Fred and gave me tour around Becca's house and told me what Becca's plan for the day was. Fred helped Becca put her clean clothes on the clothes horse and unsure of what to do, I just observed them.

Fred sensed my apprehension and encouraged me to get involved with the activities straight away. Nervously, I put on some disposable gloves and began to fold up clean pillowcases and bed sheets to go into Becca's room. Later, Fred helped Becca get out her hoover from the cupboard. *"Come on Henry, come on,"* Becca chatted happily to her hoover friend. I giggled appreciatively. Becca noticed and said I could go downstairs if I wanted. The smile was wiped off my face and I felt awkward leaving Becca up there, but as Fred was downstairs, I decided to fill in some paperwork for my induction folder.

11th November 2015

I learnt a lot about Becca on my shadowing shift today. After she tidied her house, I watched Fred supporting Becca with some money for lunch and making a list for Becca's weekly food shop. Becca told me about her hairdresser, Paul, and that she was looking forward to having purple hair with red highlights. I admire her eccentricity.

Even though I bought a packed lunch, I'd left it at Becca's house, and she wanted lunch at the pub down the road – fish finger sandwiches. I had some soup and bread roll but noticed Fred didn't have anything. It made me feel uncomfortable because I don't know if support workers are allowed to eat with the people they are supporting. Fred didn't seem too bothered.

Luckily, I could go home at 5pm.
I'm knackered.

Towards the end of November, I was coming up to completing my first month at Mencap. I was starting to get to know the people I was supporting and enjoyed shadowing some of the more independent and mildly affected residents who lived on the main road. In the last week of the month, I was given some shadowing shifts in a supported living home less than a mile away, up a big hill. I was told some of the people up there needed more support, so my new-found growing confidence for the role was beginning to evaporate.

Wednesday 25th November

It feels like I'm starting all over again. I went to a new house today so I could meet the rest of the people Mencap supports locally. I walked up this giant hill that made me think of the steep roads I've seen on tv of San Francisco. I haven't been used to walking up hills, especially after my operations and I could definitely feel my lungs having an extreme workout. I had to stop several times just to catch my breath!

Eventually I arrived at the house, just before my shift started at ten. A slim lady in her early sixties opened the door. She introduced herself as Kate and said that I would be shadowing her colleague, Sadie, today. Kate let me in, and I took in the surroundings: a small narrow hallway lay ahead of me with a flight of stairs with a stair lift and a large lounge area on the right. The walls were plastered with A4 paper scribbles and colourings as well as a large framed collage of photos of the residents.

"You're Zoë, aren't you? came a voice from upstairs. A middle-aged woman climbed into the seat of her stair lift and began to glide down towards me.

"I'm Hazel*."

"Hi, yes, I'm Zoë. Nice to meet you."

I was taken aback how friendly Hazel* was. I had just read in her support plan about her complex mood changes and occasional negative perceptions on life, but seeing her in reality, I almost couldn't believe it was the same person. I was comforted that she reminded me so much of Helen from school and that they both had a disability that impacted the way they walked and they both loved horse riding.

I was even more impressed when Sadie and I took her to the local swimming pool. As I didn't have my swimming costume, I watched how Hazel flew through the water with such strength.

Later that day I met Hazel's housemates, Callum*, who has Down's Syndrome and Daniel* who has Autism. On the last day of November, I had my induction folder signed off and I was finally able to work on my own.

Support Worker Role

As I had begun counselling training in London and was also studying a Level 3 diploma in Health and Social Care for Mencap at home, I had a twenty-hour contract to work with the Mencap residents.

I mainly worked with Callum* and became his Key Worker in the new year. I learnt all about what to include in his Support Plan when I updated it; a 'grab and run' sheet for their personal details; what their interests are, how they like to be supported; their strengths and limitations; medical details, accident forms and key worker meetings.

I worked with Callum to produce a weekly timetable that displayed what activities he did each day and who would be supporting him. Mondays were his personal day and I would observe him while he counted his weekly money allowance from his mum and supported him to buy his shopping – me pushing the trolley, him writing out his shopping list and picking up the items from the shelves. Wednesday evenings we would make the meal he had chosen from his cookbook and would often prepare a Spaghetti Carbonara or Macaroni Cheese for his housemates.

While Callum was at his day centre on a Wednesday, I would support Daniel, often known as Dan, during the day. I took over from the night staff and would support Dan with his shower and breakfast.

To maintain Dan's dignity support workers encouraged him to use the grab-rails along the walls of the house to help him walk independently and maintain muscle strength. Once Dan had used the toilet and made his way to his shower seat, I would close the plastic divider gates and check the water temperature, before talking through each step of the shower process. Staff were allowed to wash Dan's hair and his back, but we encouraged him to wash everywhere else.

While Dan dressed himself, I would prepare his breakfast – porridge with a strawberry milkshake, as well as his vast range of medication. The strangest thing was taking out his large epilepsy tablets, thinking how I had just taken smaller capsules of that very medicine with my own breakfast.

Dan was aware of his medication in his porridge. I think back to that induction training day, thankful that my peer had helped me in how to support a person with their medicine. Sometimes Dan would turn his head away, threatening a rejection of his tablets, but usually he responded well if I was calm and patient with him.

Dan was the most severely affected person at this supported living home. I learnt a lot about Autism, aware that many people with TS can be affected by it, and that Autism wasn't just some inability to be sociable or that people with Autism were devoid of any emotion. Even though they had their occasional outbursts, Dan definitely liked to joke around and tease his friends; Hazel could also talk enthusiastically on topics that interested her.

Limitations

Even though I was helpful in my role, I had to acknowledge that even I couldn't do everything. Due to my own epilepsy history, management and my colleagues agreed it was in the best interest of the people we supported and myself, that I didn't support Dan overnight. We also discussed that I felt uncomfortable with the prospect of pushing Dan and Hazel in their manual wheelchairs due to feeling sensitive about my upper body strength and the connection with my lungs - how I picked up my nephew and my lung collapsed.

Being unable to drive has also limited what I do with the people I support. Convenient five-minute drives to the shops became a two-hour round trips: walking and waiting at the bus stop and the return journey with the shopping.

But those seemingly mundane times have given me and the people I support the chance to have those in-depth conversations about the weekly discos and the social groups they go to; a chance to stop at a café for a hot chocolate, point out a friend's house or see a new film at the cinema. Even a simple walk along the river in the sunshine with an ice-cream has put a smile on their faces. It's those small moments that I can provide that still make a difference, and not only does all the exercise do my lung health good but provides regular exercise for the people I support too.

TSC and LAM Influences

If it wasn't for having TS and LAM, I probably wouldn't have chosen to work at Mencap. I wouldn't have had an interest to support adults with learning disabilities, I may not have shown Helen as much interest at school and we may not have become friends.

Working at Mencap has helped me see people with learning disabilities still matter and they want to be valued just as any other person does. I've also been able to develop my own skills in becoming an adult – managing finances, food shopping, cooking, maintaining health and safety checks; empathising with people who may seem different to me, but actually acknowledging that there are many similarities despite our differences.

The experience has helped me become more accepting of people with TS, who may have learning disabilities too.

---

*Denotes name changed to protect identity

CHAPTER 8

COUNSELLING

<u>What is Counselling?</u>

In recent years the focus on mental health has increased. However, it wasn't that long ago when issues with anxiety and depression were classed as mental breakdowns. It was, and still is in some ways, perceived as a weakness to show vulnerability – to cry or admit that you are feeling sad and troubled; that perhaps if you were to share those emotions, you could be judged as someone who needs to be in a mental institution. However, that isn't necessarily the case.

On the other hand, as I have explored in my own journey with anxiety, acknowledging our emotions gives us the permission to be human and that the more we push away how we feel, the more likely it's going to bite us back.

There is strength in vulnerability and that is gradually becoming acceptable and recognisable in society. Perhaps that is why more and more people are choosing to have counselling? But what is counselling?

Counselling is a professional therapeutic relationship between a qualified counsellor and a client. Depending on the type of therapy, weekly sessions can be short-term, six to twelve sessions or long-term, such as several years. The counsellor provides a private, non-judgemental and confidential space for the client to share their emotions and life experiences.

Rather than providing an advice service, counsellors support their clients by listening and reflecting on what their client may have said, acknowledging how they feel about an event in the past or present so they can understand themselves better. It also helps the client to feel heard and valued, particularly if they have not experienced that before.

Counselling can take many forms such as therapies in schools, colleges and universities, for children, teenagers and young adults; counselling for general mental health problems such as anxiety and depression, or specialised areas such as addiction or abuse.

Overview of counselling theories

As part of my counsellor career journey I explore different types of therapy. To begin with I experienced Cognitive Behavioural Therapy (CBT) that helps to adjust negative thought patterns into positive ones, surrounding low self-esteem or phobias. I talk about the history and background of CBT in the introduction to the chapter on Anxiety.

Person-Centred Therapy

The main theory I explore is Person-Centred Therapy which was developed in the 1950s by a psychologist called Carl Rogers (1902-1987). The American psychologist believed that every person has a need to be treated unconditionally, without judgement, to thrive as a unique human being. If we are not given that acceptance by those closest to us, including ourselves, then we lose track as to who we are as people and undermine our self-worth.

"The central truth for Rogers was that the client knows best. It is the client who knows what hurts and where the pain lies, and it is the client, who in the final analysis, will discover the way forward."

(Mearns, Thorne and McLeod, 2013)

A Person-Centred therapist supports their clients by providing, what Rogers describes as the Core Conditions: congruence (to be genuine), unconditional positive regard and empathy. Even with an unsupportive start in life, a client can learn to value in themselves.

Psychodynamic Therapy

Whereas Person-Centred therapy has a focus on events in the present, Psychodynamic therapy is based on the client looking back at past events that help them deepen their understanding of themselves.

Traditionally what is known as Psychodynamic therapy today, was more commonly referred to as Psychoanalysis in the past. Sigmund Freud (1856-1939), an Austrian-born Neurologist, would analyse how the mind works on his clients, known as patients. Initially analysing himself, he believed that the mind has three layers of awareness: the Conscious mind, the Pre-Conscious mind, and the Unconscious mind.

While the Conscious is aware of the thoughts and emotions currently in our heads, the Pre-Conscious would be an underlying layer of memories we could recall if we wanted to. These details could be things we wouldn't necessarily have to think about all the time, such as names and birthdays, whereas the Unconscious mind, the deepest layer is believed to store our most traumatic experiences. In effect these emotions could feel so painful that it seems easier to brush them aside and numb them through distractions (avoidance) as a short-term solution. Yet for some reason we might not be able to work out why we feel angry or sad about something.

It is through Psychoanalysis and Psychodynamic therapy that the therapist supports the client while they access these hidden memories and emotions, so they acknowledge and move on from these painful experiences.

Integrative Therapy

Whilst some clients may benefit from just CBT, Person-Centred or Psychodynamic therapies, other clients may find a combination of theories useful for their journey, called Integrative Counselling.

Depending on each individual, a client may find an Integrative therapist useful because they may want the empathic, non-judgemental approach from a Person-Centred counsellor, but want to explore their childhood trauma from the past. As part of my Integrative Counselling training, I explored a wider range of therapeutic approaches but mainly found the combination of Person-Centred and Psychodynamic theories most helpful in understanding my TS/ LAM experiences which have helped me to write this book.

The Tavistock and Portman NHS Trust

The start of my counselling career journey began at the Tavistock and Portman NHS Trust. The organisation began as two separate bodies. The Tavistock Clinic was set up in 1920 for soldiers in the First World War who had suffered from Post-Traumatic Stress Disorder (PTSD) and The Portman Clinic established in 1931 for patients involved with criminal acts of violence. In 1948, the National Health Service (NHS) became a part of The Tavistock Clinic to support people with mental health issues and developed training courses for mental health professionals. By 1994, the two clinics joined together to form the Tavistock and Portman NHS Trust.

My Experience

24th September 2015

I enrolled at the Tavistock and Portman NHS Trust centre today. It was good to be back in London and there was a real excitement in the air about a new start.

After enrolling, I walked along to the Freud Museum, which was set in the house he used to live in when he moved to England. It was really interesting. I had a ham and cheese panini in a café for lunch.

While I was eating, I had some time to reflect on the photography degree I achieved the previous year and how since then I had changed careers. I thought back to my almost-constant interest in the mind and personality growing up; my enjoyment of listening and understanding people; going on my own therapeutic journey of CBT to overcome anxiety, before riding the turbulent waves of ill health with TS and LAM.

I had to go through all that to decide I wanted to become a counsellor...?

Memories of 2013 seemed tough. The tight belt of tension around my abdomen was becoming unbearable, I was tired of struggling and I knew I had to surrender and ask for professional help. But I didn't know anything about therapy.

Am I going to be sat on one of those long sofas and be given advice that will magically fix my problems?

When I had Cognitive Behavioural Therapy, I was surprised that therapy wasn't about being given advice, that there isn't one solution for everyone. Although I had weekly telephone support from my therapist, I discovered that a lot of the therapeutic process was done when I was alone. I gained an understanding of where my fears came from and ways to overcome it. I merely discussed my insights with my therapist.

I found being a client beneficial too, but I liked the idea of being a therapist for someone as well, supporting them with their issues. It was during that time I warmed to the prospect of becoming a counsellor, but I was only half-way through my photography degree.

Six months after my therapy had finished, I managed to pluck the courage to discuss with my parents that I wasn't going to follow-through with becoming a professional photographer. I also had the support of Vivien, a family friend, who had changed careers and became a counsellor as well. She had heard the Tavistock and Portman NHS Trust do some introductory courses, and I may find them useful.

2015

The course I enrolled for was an *Introduction to Counselling and Psychotherapy* that described itself as being *suitable* for people wanting to begin their counselling career. It was a perfect fit.

29th September 2015

Today I had my first lecture at the Tavistock. It was strange getting the train and how I thought my studying time in London was over. Apart from the enrolment day, the last time I was in London I was in hospital – a cannula in my hand and a chest drain in my side. It was just over year ago I had the very first chest drain put in for my left lung. It's been a lot to take in.

I wrote in great detail that evening about how despite my nerves of being in a new class, I was fascinated by all the topics I would be learning about; understanding what Psychotherapy is and all its fancy terms; human development and the varying types of mental health from Depression to Psychosis. I was never as excited about photography theory as I was about this.

Over the following months I was able to start my Support Worker job for Mencap and use my role as part of a work placement in a helping environment. Not only was I able to develop my skills in working with adults with learning disabilities, but I could also refer to the knowledge I was absorbing about mental health.

2016

As the new year came around, I was not only learning about theory, but I was also gaining insight as well.

23rd February 2016

It was interesting to learn in class about how people respond to stress by using common defence mechanisms. I had used avoidance to resist my anxiety, but I only became aware of that through having therapy.

My lecturer also mentioned that if we continue further training, it's beneficial to see a counsellor for our own development. She said it would help us become aware of our hidden thoughts, but that sounds really scary. It's amazing when people are able to do that. But I've sorted through my anxiety… so, what would I talk about?

A few weeks later, we looked at difference and diversity in class. Some peers shared their experiences, but I held back. I silently reflected over how I've always felt different growing up. I saw it as: I have TS and everyone else doesn't…but then there are other people who have TS, but I'm not like them either.

15ᵗʰ March 2016

Maybe I'm trying to differentiate myself from TS people. Maybe that is making me feel more isolated? I probably relate to non-TS people more, but then they don't know what it's like to live with it. I wish I wasn't so uncertain about other TS people. Am I afraid of them? Am I scared to admit I have it?

For a while I remained confused. I was confused about what kind of therapist I wanted to be; whether I still wanted to be a CBT therapist or a Psychotherapist, and I was confused about myself and where I fitted in. By mid-May, the year-long course had come to an end.

17ᵗʰ May 2016

Endings. That was the theme for our last lesson. Endings mean different things to different people. Endings can be sad, like when Granny died, or endings can be happy. I was so relieved to be discharged from hospital when my lungs were finally secure.

I hadn't really considered the end of this course until now. This ending is a loss of something familiar and this course has been familiar to me in the past year. I imagine I'm going to continue my training, but the next course focuses on psychiatric hospitals and I don't want to work in one of those. It's why we all hate change so much. Uncertainty of the future, a potential loss, but it's a chance to try again and start a new chapter. I began thinking about this after my appointment at the LAM centre last week and that I'm coming to terms with having it. It's been like a mourning period. A loss of an idealised image of my perfect health. I know with TS, my health was never 100% perfect, but it's been fairly strong overall. Discovering I have LAM has been like starting all over again and facing the truth that I will always have both conditions. I've just been trying to adjust to it.

Counselling Part 2: Self-Acceptance

Over the summer months I spoke to our family friend, Vivien, about my potential next steps in becoming a counsellor. In the autumn, I stumbled across the Counselling and Psychotherapy Training Academy (CPTA) who provide further training across the UK, with a centre local to me.

I looked at the Level 2 course that focussed on developing counselling skills for people working in helping environments. Having worked for Mencap for almost a year and since I had completed my introductory certificate at the Tavistock, this was great.

Over the next two years, I completed the Level 2 course and the Level 3 diploma, deepening my understanding of mental health and self-awareness.

2018

Getting on to the Level 4 diploma was an achievement. If I could complete the next two years, I could become a qualified counsellor. However, in order to get to that goal post, I would not only have to complete a counselling placement, but also have my own therapy sessions too.

October

A month into my course and I had found a counsellor who lived a short distance away. She worked in a Person-Centred therapeutic approach that my course prioritised; face-to-face sessions that focused on what the client wanted to discuss rather than solution-based therapy such as CBT.

Upon the arrival of my initial meeting session, I was filled with mixed feelings; excited but nervous; wondering why I was having counselling, as I didn't need it like I did for anxiety. I knocked on my counsellor's door and we introduced ourselves, before letting me in. I slipped off my shoes and followed Catherine into the counselling room. I sat on the sofa opposite her. I felt comfortable and relaxed.

At first it was as I expected, going through the contract details on how we were going to work together, but then I came across the page in the contract that mentioned *health*.

My calm, tranquil state disappeared, and I felt sick as I read questions in front of me about health conditions and medical and emergency contact details. Questions I hated answering the most.

Avoiding eye contact, I took a breath and swallowed down my nerves, before writing down the words *Tuberous Sclerosis, Epilepsy* and *LAM*. After filling in the remainder of the contract, I signed the bottom of the agreement and handed it back.

As part of the Person-Centred approach, Catherine wanted to find out who I was as a person, so she would know how to support me throughout the course. I hadn't been expecting to say the names of my conditions out loud and what they involve, in addition to writing them down. Other than medical professionals, teachers and family, only a handful of people knew what my conditions were called and how they worked. To tell someone I had only just met never happened.

12th October 2018

I'm amazed how open I was in sharing such personal information for my first counselling session. Not only did I discuss TS and LAM, but my counsellor noticed that although my conditions have an invisible element to them, they have impacted me on quite an emotional level; my shyness growing up and how I have been selective in who I trust.

The following week, we met for our second session. Feeling brave, I continued to talk about my life, but when I mentioned my health, I carefully avoided saying the words TS and LAM.

"I notice you say, 'my health conditions' rather than their names."

"Err, yeah...it's just that one of them sounds like another condition (Tuberculosis) *and I don't want people to get confused, because no one has really heard of mine."*

My answer was accepted, but it felt to me like a lucky escape. The following day I reflected over the session.

20th October 2018

I admit that to some extent, I do run away from TS-related topics. We discussed how I'm more accepting of myself externally but it's the internal (emotional/physical) elements that I'm most sensitive about – the experiences I've been through, that I haven't really spoken about those in much detail yet.

We agreed that I've probably created a barrier between the outside me, who is 'condition-free', with the hidden internal self, who is afraid of getting too close to people in case they don't accept all of me.

We explored in my session that perhaps it's less about wanting to be accepted by others, but more about self-acceptance. Learning to acknowledge the parts of me I find difficult to, not just the parts of me that are easy to live with.

I don't want to run away from myself, my emotions or my thoughts. I know all this counselling will feel uncomfortable as I face myself, but that's part of the process.

21st October 2018

The more prepared I am to be myself and accept all of me, the less ashamed I will feel about being someone with two health conditions. I think I have to accept what I've been through with TS and LAM, rather than pretending they don't exist. At the moment, the only time I really acknowledge them is when I have my hospital appointments.

I've been through some awful experiences but despite them I have got through them and become healthier. I may be limited in what I can do, but there is still so much that I can achieve.

November

It was a few more weeks before I had any more sessions due to school holidays and a hospital appointment. I had an EEG scan to monitor the electrical waves in my brain after having my first Focal Aware seizure in two months a few days before. I was filled with disappointment.

9th November 2018

In therapy today I opened up about how disappointed I felt about my epilepsy and the negative thoughts it brings. I spoke about the denial, and we agreed that accepting TS and LAM like I did for Anxiety seems like the best approach forward. I didn't have to like having health conditions, but acknowledging they are there is ok.

Since I began my counselling training, Vivien had given me many of the books that helped her through her own studying. One of the books was about making sense of emotions through drawing. After my session, I got the book and my sketchbook out and drew three pictures of me on a page – Child Me, Teenage Me and Adult Me.

Child Me was surrounded by happy and positive words to describe herself. Teenage Me was surrounded by words depicting insecurity and doubt, and Adult me was a mixture of the two. The combination of positive and negative descriptions was like the happy and unhappy parts of me coming together.

Child Me, representing a time before I was truly aware I had TS and I could express myself in a colourful, free, way. Approaching adolescence, I struggled with not being like everyone else and this is where those defence mechanisms came into play – the start of that denial as a way of coping. Then Adult Me, beginning to acknowledge TS and LAM; the low confidence of my past with its physical and emotional hurdles, but revisiting the colourful child inside that I had abandoned.

I realised that I'm not just someone 'normal' (condition-free) and I'm not just someone who is completely TS and LAM. I'm a combination of both.

December

Due to a common side effect of my lung medication, I caught an infection under my arm and I had minor surgery to remove it. Emotionally and physically, I was taken back to those times of intense pain and recuperation, as well as anxieties of uncertainty and confusion. I was supposed to be accepting TS and LAM, but this experience was challenging that.

9th December 2018

I had my dressing changed at the walk-in clinic this morning. The nurse said it will still be a while before the wound site has healed and that has got me down. It's like I'm not making any progress, even though I am. It's just really slow and I'm frustrated.

In the week before Christmas my wound no longer needed a dressing, and I was able to attend my choir's Christmas annual meet-up. Despite my recent operation, I was seeing a development in my confidence and my choir friends could see it too. Maybe I was beginning to accept myself after all?

2019

Over the next six months, I discussed in therapy the boundaries that I had subconsciously put up against the world. I wanted to connect with people who also have TS and LAM, but I felt guilty that I didn't want to either.

8th July 2019

I've just finished the first year of my Level 4 counselling diploma. I've started working with my first clients on a placement at a sixth form college and I've had twenty-six counselling sessions since October.

I never expected to talk about my health conditions so openly in my personal counselling sessions, but I've learnt so much from doing so. I was able to start facing the emotional side I had been hiding from for so long.

Everyone has aspects of themselves that they initially disapprove of but it's only by working through those, rather than covering them up or repressing them that helps to develop self-acceptance.

It doesn't mean to say though that it's been easy; the emotional discomfort has been tough sometimes. It's much easier to numb and distract yourself, but I've realised those aspects will always be there no matter how hard I would try to bat them away.

Rather than seeing TS and LAM as just the negative side of me and everything else as normal and positive, I've been able to combine the two. I remember drawing pictures of myself at different stages but really, it's much easier to view that thought process as a Venn diagram. It's where those two conflicting circles of negativity and positivity when overlapped, create the balanced me who feels whole and content with who she is.

The one who can acknowledge she isn't all bad and isn't all good either, but human and real. It's an amazing feeling to have, and has been great to discuss that in therapy.

After my realisation, I felt like I was living on a new baseline, that as long as I acknowledged all aspects of myself, then I could be happy... but I couldn't discount that now I had reached this self-acceptance goal post, that it was a bit lonely being at the top of a metaphorical mountain on my own. What was I going to do now?

September

When the second year of my diploma began, I resumed my counselling sessions. I described how although I had gained self-acceptance, I still felt lost. I was encouraged to elaborate.

13th September 2019

It's a bit like standing on the outskirts of a forest. I love trees and I feel calm and content around them, but I can't see where the path is going. It disappears into the woods, where dark shadows cover up the uneven ground, but in some places, there is sunlight trying to come through the trees...

My metaphor was a reminder of how despite feeling whole in myself, life would still have its ups and downs. Only by walking into the forest and following my path was I going to find out. I was reminded of Brené Brown's book *Braving the Wilderness*. This was my wilderness.

November

Towards the end of the month I was regaining my confidence and entered some photos in the village Arts and Crafts exhibition. The 2019 theme was Masks: I had two halves to my photo; the left side of the image – a full length self-portrait of me in a long dress hidden behind a Venetian mask, and on the right a casual portrait of me in a plain t-shirt and jogging bottoms without my mask. Through this, I was able to reflect over my self-acceptance journey in the past year. I shared this on my blog.

20th November 2019

Masks are fascinating in many ways. A mask can be a physical object that covers the face, or it can be an emotional mask where we hide our feelings and personality behind it. Make-up for example, can be a way of concealing who we really are.

I've never been one for much make-up, but for a long time I wore an emotional mask and felt insecure about having two rare health conditions. I wasn't happy in my own skin.

Through having personal counselling alongside my own counselling training, I came to terms with my situation and I was a lot more accepting of my beautiful, imperfect self. This project is a visual chance to show how I don't have to wear any kind of mask anymore, and that it so freeing. Yes, it can feel uncomfortable to begin with, but what are we really afraid of?

People who are brave enough to reveal their authentic selves are far more beautiful because they light up from within; that no amount of material items, layers of foundation or false eye lashes can ever buy that.

Yes, masks can be scary; they can be scary to look at or even be scary to hide behind. We want to believe in the façade that our lives are perfect, but even in the best circumstances, no one's life is, no one is flawless.

2020

February

After my counselling exams were out of the way in January, the first week in February meant a presentation in front of my peers on Difference and Diversity. Fortunately, the presentation was a group project, and being paired with the only man on the course gave us both a varied understanding on what Difference and Diversity meant for each of us.

We agreed on a quote on diversity that we shared with the class:

"The concept of diversity encompasses acceptance and respect. It means understanding each individual is unique and recognising our individual differences. This includes race, ethnicity, gender, sexual orientation, socioeconomic status, age, physical abilities, religious beliefs or other ideologies"

(Queensborough Community College)

Before we opened up the topic of what difference and diversity meant for the rest of the class, I shared my own personal experience:

For me I am affected by a rare genetic health condition called Tuberous Sclerosis Complex. It's a condition I was born with that affects "1 million people worldwide". It involves benign tumours that can grow on key organs such as the skin, brain, heart, lungs and kidneys, which can vary from person to person. This depends on the location and size of the tumours.

For example, many people with the condition may have physical or learning disabilities, while others may not know they have TS at all.

For me TS has mainly affected my confidence in society and has caused me to experience epilepsy from a young age, as well as operations on my lungs and my right kidney in my early twenties.

But because of my experiences it has made me more accepting of other people who identify with feeling different too and has influenced my career path as a Support Worker for Mencap and becoming a counsellor.

After the class discussions and the main presentation, people from my class and my teachers came up to me throughout the day saying how brave I was to share such personal information about myself, and that they had no idea. I responded with half-awkward-smiles and thanks, but I don't think my peers realised how much their praise meant to me.

For the rest of the month I was digesting the experience of telling my class about myself and how I would have never done that four years ago on my introductory course at the Tavistock.

*

By March, it was good to discover that my diverse diploma class had all passed our exams, and we could all celebrate our achievement together; cheering and giving out hugs and high-fives. Although we had some way to go with completing final assignments and client hours on placement, I definitely felt a sense of self-acceptance and a positive change in the way I view others who have the conditions that I have too.

CHAPTER 9

GETTING INVOLVED WITH THE TSA

What is the Tuberous Sclerosis Association (TSA)

The Tuberous Sclerosis Association is the leading charity in the UK, supporting people and their families with Tuberous Sclerosis Complex (TSC). The organisation was set up in 1977, when three women (Ann Hunt, Jean Wilson and Ester Galbraith) discovered they all had children with TSC, and they decided to write letters to each other. Together they founded the organisation and the TSA officially became a registered charity in 1978.

In the same year a regular newsletter called Scan was sent around the country to other families who were affected by TSC, and as the charity grew, the newsletter became a magazine, which continues to be delivered to TSC families four times a year.

Throughout the 1980s and 1990s funding for TSC research was being developed. The unknown disease was gradually growing in awareness and between 1993-1997, the two genes behind the disease, TSC1 and TSC2 had been discovered. National TSC clinics were also being opened in hospitals around the country at the turn of 21st century.

Support Groups

In the midst of breakthrough research developments, members of the TSC community set up a support group called Outlook, for mildly affected adults. The first annual meeting took place in 1996. Outlook continues to run and celebrated their 20th anniversary in 2016.

Family Fun Days, set up in 1987, also provide additional opportunities for the wider TSC community to share their experiences. What began with *McDonalds* parties in the 1990s has grown into day trips to the seaside, farms and zoos.

My Experiences:

McDonalds Meetings

When I think of *McDonalds,* I think of vibrant fizzy drinks in a paper cup with a bendy plastic straw. I have a *Happy Meal* box next to my drink, filled with chicken nuggets, salty twiggy chips and a plastic toy. I remember the birthday parties and family days out where we would have a *McDonalds* meal for lunch or dinner treat. They were hazy but positive memories...

2002

When I turned nine things were changing. Sarah was eighteen and moved out to live at university. Geoffrey was twenty, he also moved out. I felt sadness, confusion and emptiness that my playtime buddies had left me. All my other friends had their siblings around. Why did I have to be any different?

With an ample reflection time now on my hands, I thought back over the past year and how my parents told me about having TS and me wanting to reject everything about it. My sunny relationship with *McDonalds* was about to change too when the Tuberous Sclerosis Association (TSA) invited TS-affected families to their 25th Anniversary events around the country. Our local event was at a *McDonalds* in Oxford. Reluctantly I went along with my parents, sitting in the car with a heavy frown and a turned-down mouth; my arms crossed grumpily over my chest.

When we arrived, the greasy smell of the restaurant unpleasantly filled my nose, and the sticky floor squelched against the soles of my shoes. I walked alongside Mum and Dad to the large group of TS-families, of many ages and abilities. This whole concept felt alien to me. The lighting in the restaurant was glaringly bright, yet the tables we were shown to were in a more darkly lit corner. I felt surrounded by blindingly red t-shirts that read TS in big white scary letters and *Tuberous Sclerosis* in smaller text next to it. My face scrunched up in disgust as I uncomfortably observed my surroundings; a strange mixture of loud, cheerful yet painful wails, and a blur of animated voices.

Urgh! Those red t-shirts! Those letters staring at me in the face reminding me of what I've got! All these strange people...I'm not like THEM! They have TS way worse than I do! I don't want TS. I hate being at this party. I hate my red bumpy face. They've all got red blotchy faces too...my school friends don't get to waste their Saturday at some party they don't want to be at. When can I go home....?

The rest of the event remained a blur, with only a small glow of happiness filling me up when I received a 75 pack of *Crayola* crayons to take home. A big wide smile spread across my face. *Finally, this party has something worthwhile about it.*

Relieved and mildly contented, everyone said their goodbyes and I swung my box of crayons by its big yellow handle as Mum, Dad and I walked back to the car. I plugged myself into my portable CD player and let my weary mind wander to the sounds of S Club 7.

The Intermediate Years

No way was I going to attend one of those TS meetings ever again. It was uncomfortable enough looking TS in the face at my hospital appointments in Bath, I didn't have to look at it any other time if I didn't want to.

Other than those appointment days, I shoved TS into the dark depths of my mind. When those days did come by, I was emotional, grumpy and withdrawn. For the rest of the year, I could just be Zoë – someone who doesn't have to acknowledge TS and can just go about her day like any normal person.

The following year in 2003, my epilepsy activity was re-activated; more of TS to acknowledge on a regular basis. By 2008, I had been on epilepsy medication for five years and came off it for a while, now I was fifteen. I celebrated with my favourite blackcurrant alcoholic drink mixed with lemonade.

As I approached eighteen in 2011, anxiety around my health was eating away at me, wearing down my immune system. While suffering from Bronchitis I also began showing the early signs of TS-related LAM through minor lung collapses and a kidney bleed in 2013.

Towards the end of that year, I felt motivated to contribute my anxiety journey on my favourite wellbeing blog called *Tiny Buddha*. I was inspired how people all over the world shared their life experiences and that provided hope for others. I felt with my story, I could do the same.

Articles & Volunteering

<u>2014</u>

In April my *Tiny Buddha* article was published online, and I felt a wave of achievement fill me up. I received comments from other readers who described their similar mental health experiences and felt a sense of community and respect from sharing my vulnerability that was benefitting other people.

Despite years of emotionally separating myself from TS, I began to consider whether writing about my recent health experiences would have a similar benefit to the TS community. There was a Share Your Story section of the TSA website. *I could do that. I could inspire other people and get my story published in the Scan magazine.*

21ˢᵗ April 2014

I have just finished writing my story. I wrote about my diagnosis; how I'm affected by TS; my epilepsy, the kidney bleed, and my anxiety journey. I spoke about how I'm a normal person who just happens to have the condition. It's helped me empathise with other minority groups and I believe in myself more. Despite feeling different growing up, I've been given the opportunity to be myself and feel less pressure to follow the crowd and do what everyone else is doing. I imagine that's quite a rare thing. I could use my normality to create a bridge from TS people to non-TS people. The feeling of fulfilment sending off my story is amazing. I just hope it inspires.

Although I received a confirmation email that my story had been received, my confidence of it being published dwindled every time a new issue of Scan came through the post. In the following months I busied myself with completing my final projects for university and considered applying to be a Volunteer Photographer for the TSA. A week before graduation, I filled in my TS volunteer form and sent it to the Volunteer Coordinator, Tanya. By the end of August, I finally had a Photography Degree and I officially became a volunteer for the TSA.

September

After the volunteer safeguarding checks, Dad and I attended my first volunteer placement: the TSA Staff Day. Our job was to take portraits of the staff that would be featured at the back of each Scan magazine.

12*th* September 2014

I had an exciting day. I was a little nervous about taking photos, but I was glad Dad was there to set up the white background and the lights. I was surprised how many of the staff said they didn't usually like having their photos taken, but somehow that openness made taking their photos a bit easier. They had insecurities too.

Whereas I usually feel most comfortable taking photos of inanimate objects, I was proud of myself for talking to a group of new people and capturing their faces. Before the Staff Day I had ordered myself a purple t-shirt with the latest TS logo. The purple tone made me feel calmer than that bright, glary red, and although the font was still white, the typeface was in a gentle, soft lower-case layout *"tsa: tuberous sclerosis association"*. Much more friendly. I was thinking how I could get used to this volunteering. This could be fun.

Four days later, I had my first major lung collapse.

The next seven months dragged on for what felt like an eternity. Intense shoulder pain, breathlessness; chest drains being inserted into my sides. Stress. Fatigue. Operations, and hours that passed heavily as I recovered in my aching body and chest, from the discomfort of unfamiliar hospital beds.

But before 2014 came to a close, I was greeted with an unexpected hope from the TS Scan Magazine.

11th December 2014

Just had an email from Isobel, the editor of Scan. Apparently, the TSA forwarded my email to her and could she contact me about a telephone interview. She wants to ask me about what it's like to live with TS and be involved in article about how I came to volunteer for the TSA. This sounds amazing!

Finally, despite recent emotional and physical pain, something in my life to do with TS was positive. I had been waiting for months on end to get my article published but this was even better. This wasn't just about having TS, it was about my volunteering too.

15th December 2014

Today was the day I had my interview over the phone with Isobel. She was really lovely, but I was embarrassed that my voice was all croaky. I guess I haven't done much talking since my op – or perhaps it's a chest infection? She asked me questions about my experience with TS and what inspired me to volunteer. She then sent a draft article of what will be put in the magazine. I need to get some pictures together to go alongside it.

2015

Less than a week after the New Year, I heard back from Isobel.

5th January 2015

Something staggeringly amazing happened today. Just before I went on a walk, I saw the email in my inbox. I didn't want to deal with it straight away, so I went out first. Walking down a muddy lane, I imagined what Isobel might have said. I envisaged myself on the front of Scan with my camera and how cool that would be...

NO WAY! That was exactly what she requested!

The shock and excitement I felt resonated with what only I can describe as Mike Wazowski's reaction when he discovers he is on the front of the Monsters Inc magazine. Disbelief mixed with excitement.

The following day, when the Christmas decorations had been packed away in the cupboards, Dad and I set up the white backdrop, before I changed into some jeans, my purple charity t-shirt and put on my new *inner hope* necklace. As Dad took my picture, he noticed that the white TS logo on the magazine wouldn't be seen on the front cover if the main photo background was white too.

We reconsidered and decided for me to sit on the stairs in the hallway, with me holding his camera, while he took my photo with mine. When we were happy, we sent the final selection for Isobel to choose from.

February

Almost two weeks after visiting the National LAM Centre in Nottingham and coming to terms with the realities of TS-related LAM, it was a relief to see my smiling face pop through the letter box; the shiny Scan spring issue cover. *Zoë Bull: TSA Volunteer.* I was beaming. Instantly I flicked through the magazine to the double-page-spread. Page 10. *Zoë Bull: Volunteering for the TSA.*

> "*Having lived most of her 21 years relatively free from TS symptoms, Zoë Bull has spent much of the last two years dealing with kidney and lung problems related to her TS. It was these recent experiences along with a desire to meet other affected people and to make a positive personal contribution to the TS community, which led her, a few months back, to click on the Volunteering Pages on the TSA website...*"

(SCAN Spring Issue 2015)

As I read the rest of Isobel's words in the article, I couldn't help but smile and shake my head that an article about me had just been delivered through my door and to other TS-affected families all over the UK.

Once I read the article text, I studied the photos that I had chosen with my family to be added. A smaller version of the front cover image smiled back at me; a wide grinned portrait of me at Wembley Stadium from the previous July, dressed head to toe in my blue sundress – the mortarboard and gown, arms outstretched to the sides. A large photo on the right-hand page of me in my favourite hoody, holding two flimsy L-plate stickers from 2012 that I no longer needed; and at the bottom, an image of me lying on an elevated hospital bed, with a yellow-toned complexion in a saggy hospital gown. My expression in the photo distant and exhausted. The emotional pain hit me hard as I stared uncomfortably at the state I had been in. It was the day after my kidney embolisation two-and-a-half years ago. How far I had come since then...

I was able to share my achievements with my friends, neighbours and family, who gave me their support and their pride. Later that week I showed my magazine article to Dr Amin at my routine check-up in Bath who said that his TS patients would really like this. It was more than I ever expected.

March

Despite having secured a volunteer role at the TSA and my article published, I couldn't ignore much longer that I needed to find a paid job as well. I applied to various places, none of which were successful.

16th March 2015

My emotions were all over the place today. The tough act of finding a job made me cry out of the blue and Mum could see

*how hard this was for me. Dad agreed I should just keep
searching and that I'm doing the best that I can.*

*The TSA Volunteer Manager emailed me about a postcard
campaign that she thought I might be interested in. The photo
on the front is supposed to represent what it's like to have TS
with a short paragraph on the back about the experience. At
least it's something positive I can focus on.*

Over the next week, motivation for my job search returned
and I applied for a Support Worker role at Mencap. Although
hopeful, my confidence was still low.

<u>22nd March 2015</u>

*I have been worried about people finding out about TS
because I look so normal on the outside. Sometimes it's like
I'm an imposter who is not deserving of being normal. But
when people found out about it through my article, they were
so accepting.*

After writing yesterday's journal post, I was inspired to create
the photo for the postcard campaign. I went downstairs and
picked up two small models of a white sheep and a black
sheep from a noughts and crosses set and brought them up to
my room. I took all the items off my bedside table and put
them on the floor. With a clear space, I placed a thick 7x8 glass
panel from a photo frame I had got for Christmas onto the
wooden table and positioned the two sheep models either side
of the glass, staring at each other.

After taking some photos, I uploaded them onto my computer
and studied what I had just created. A white sheep looking at
its reflection with a black sheep staring back. I gazed out of the
window, wincing at the rawness of emotion I had just
acknowledged.

Is this how I really think of myself?

It perfectly described my seemingly external normality yet how I saw myself internally. My family and friends appreciated me unconditionally, so why couldn't I?

In a Word document, I wrote a large paragraph outlining my TS and LAM journey so far for the postcard. I described the shyness I developed in childhood, self-conscious about the red, bumpy, facial fibromas on my nose and cheeks. I added an excerpt from that journal post, that was going to be placed next to the photo of the sheep.

I have been worried about people finding out about TS because I look so normal on the outside

When I was happy with my creation, I sent the image and the text to the TSA. A few months later I received my own postcard in the post, proud of my achievement, hoping it would help raise awareness with the other postcards the TS community had made.

April

Although I was over the moon that I had been offered the Support Worker role at Mencap, my excited reaction caused my right lung to collapse when I jumped up and down. *This just isn't fair.*

The first week of April was full of tests, oxygen masks and needles. My lung inflated but afterwards the medical team agreed that it would be a good idea to have a planned operation on my lung so it wouldn't collapse again. I knew it would be the safest long-term option for me but agreeing felt like a defeat that I wasn't ready to face.

With the operation due at the end of April, I was able to return home. I enjoyed my twenty-second birthday with all my family, and then several days later I gathered all my physical and emotional strength to attend my first TSA Outlook event.

My First Outlook Event

It was a fresh, spring morning and Mum and Dad drove me up to Birmingham where Outlook was being held. I plugged myself into my iPod and let my thoughts drift tirelessly around my brain. Not writing anything in my journal that day made me realise how emotionally testing this was for me.

I hadn't met anyone with TS for social reasons since that *McDonald's* party. I knew I had been dismissive and didn't feel like them. Yet having overcome a kidney bleed and both lungs collapsing, I perhaps could relate to the TS community more than ever.

The following day, I was able to collect my thoughts enough to write them down.

19th April 2015

When I arrived at the hotel, butterflies were starting to flutter in my stomach. I stepped into a small lounge area in the lobby where people were chatting away. Once I spotted a TSA staff member, she introduced me to a fashion degree student called Tim*. He seemed mildly affected by TS too and I felt my insecurities about being accepted fall way. I spoke so freely to Tim and his mum and explained that I had never really spoken to anyone with TS before.

Before the main conference started, a young woman called Natalie* exchanged smiles with me. Suddenly we were sitting next to each other talking about having TS and how we both had varying degrees of epilepsy.

One of the events in the day was from a mindfulness teacher. I've done a bit of mindfulness for my anxiety, so it's been helpful to revisit it. We were asked to write down two things we find challenging about living with TS; and what we are grateful for. I noted down I hated unexpected change but that I was grateful that non-TS people wanted to invest their time researching this rare condition that I otherwise wouldn't know about.

After the exercise we all shared our thoughts. It gave me a sense of how people in Outlook have been affected. How some have struggled with their education, while others have been to university or work for the NHS; the prejudice people had felt and how someone said it bothered them when Tuberous Sclerosis was misheard as Tuberculosis. I laughed to myself, as that was the very reason, I didn't like telling people the name of the condition.

At lunchtime I met some new faces, initiating conversations... ME? I felt fantastic and free. I spoke to another young woman who lived in West London, near where I went to university. We talked about our strengths and weaknesses at school concerning TS.

When the afternoon session started, we all got a chance to mingle with other people. I spoke to parents of grown-up children with TS who were coming to Outlook for the first time, and those with carers. Original Outlook members came over and offered any advice they had. Their attitude was warm and friendly, yet I felt a bit swamped when I was handed their contact details straightaway – I had only just met them.

I felt a bit sensitive stretching my arms out after my time in hospital recently when we did some yoga exercises, but I felt grounded as I planted my feet firmly to the floor. The position was called Mountain Pose and we had to imagine being strong and powerful – that we can think ourselves into positivity as we can think ourselves into negativity. The beauty of it was that it was relatively easy for everyone to join in.

At the end of the day the large group of us sat on the floor in a circle, discussing the 2016 Outlook event with the TSA Chairman. As he was talking, I looked around the group. There was such a range of people: young adults to those in their early sixties; an array of skin tones and cultures; those who had mild autism and learning difficulties to vision impairments, and members who just had the odd element here and there like the facial fibromas and the white ash leaf skin patches…

I enjoyed myself, yet I couldn't help still feeling different from this group. But why? I let my guard down and made some connections. There were people of similar abilities to me; we all had TS…I could be myself, and not pretend I was condition-free. I didn't have to worry whether they would accept me. *Isn't that what I want? Was I going to attend next year's Outlook? Did I want to?*

Although I didn't know it at the time, I was subconsciously being reminded of the emotional discomfort I faced at the *McDonalds* party. I didn't want to have anything to do with TS. I didn't want to relate to anyone more severely affected than me. But at the present time, I had just met a whole group of people who did seem mildly affected, relatively normal. Friendly. Although I belonged, I still felt lost.

*

Despite my confusion, I felt a familiar spark inside that I had got when I decided to write my story for Scan; *I could write an article about my first experience at Outlook to encourage more people like me to come along.*

The next day I contacted Isobel who agreed it would be a great idea and that she would rearrange the Outlook section of the magazine to fit my article in. Wow! I couldn't believe it. I was going to have another article in the next Scan issue. My second consecutive publication in the magazine.

Spring into Summer

At the end of April, I had my planned operation to secure my right lung to my chest wall. After spending half of May in hospital, the summer was about recuperating. While I was recovering physically, I was at war with myself emotionally.

19th June 2015

My mind is a blur. I don't know what I'm doing. I'm trying to make sense of...I don't know, even thinking just seems like an effort. I feel I'm trying to be perfect in some way and there is some underlying insecurity. I have told myself that I need to be strong, emotionally and physically. I know I'm healing. Maybe I'm just impatient? I feel lost and I want to trust my body. I worry about the future and what is going on inside me. I need to be patient and kind to my wellbeing.

24ᵗʰ July 2015

I know I'm insecure, but the best thing for me to do is to accept myself. I may not have full control over TS and LAM, but I'm on medication and I can control my thoughts. If I can change how I perceive anxiety, I can change how I see myself. I can't hide from myself forever.

9ᵗʰ August 2015

I'm still in conflict with myself, but I received an email newsletter from my favourite magazine about learning to like who we are. I clicked the link to the video and listened to a lady who said when we accept ourselves, we neither obsess nor dislike who we are. We become ok with how our bodies are right now rather than what we want them to be. I can't change that I have TS and LAM, but I could accept that I have both conditions and that currently, although I'm healing, I'm stable and healthy. I like how she said there said there are no rules on how to be – that we can look, dress and do what we want, rather than being a certain way to fit in. It was like this video was giving me the permission to be my true self, something I rarely felt I could do unless I was with my family or closest friends.

September

It was glad to see the summer come to end and that some new beginnings were on the horizon. My application for Mencap had been resumed, I was about to start my counselling training, and my second nephew was due to be born that month.

I was feeling emotionally and physically stronger than I had done since April, and I had agreed in May to take some photos for a TS science and research event in mid-September.

11th September 2015

It was the last day of the science conference in Windsor. It was rainy and I was full of adrenaline; slotting in some meditation before breakfast. I listened to a relaxing playlist as I got dressed into my purple TSA t-shirt. Looking in the mirror was like facing up to the part of me I like to hide. I turned away from my reflection.

I was pleased to have Dad supporting me at the event. The conference room was dark, but I could see the slides illuminated on the wall from where I was standing. The information was very academic, and it was quite overwhelming to take in, seeing as I had been through quite a lot recently.

I was relieved when the presentation was over as I was able to take some candid photos of medical professionals and scientists socialising over the buffet. One lady noticed my purple t-shirt and asked where she could get one. I gave her

RARE: A JOURNEY OF SELF-ACCEPTANCE

the details and she said thanks, but what I appreciated most, was that she remembered my face from the Scan magazine cover, and that I really inspired her.

End of year summary

It was a great feeling to have inspired someone and I left the event feeling I had done some good. At the end of the year, I received an email with a report from the TSA over 2015. I was amazed to see a summarised article of my voluntary work that I had done with the three photos included in my SCAN story back in the spring. A few days later I received a certificate celebrating my first year of volunteering for the TSA. I felt really proud.

The Outlook 20th Anniversary

2016

As 2016 came into view, I was almost halfway through my introductory counselling course in London and became a Key Worker for a man with Down's Syndrome at Mencap. My health was looking better, and I was being introduced to a new medication to help support both my TS and LAM. In terms of the TSA, the Outlook group was going to be celebrating its 20th anniversary in April with a 1920s themed evening.

February

8th February 2016

Stormy. Windy. Wet. Cold. On the way to work, I decided to go into the hat shop I've walked past many times. I saw a brown cloche that would be perfect with my sage green 1920s dress. I loved the little bell that rang as I went through the door and was amazed the hat was on sale at £55.00 down from £215.00. I could treat myself to that.

Over the next few months I received the schedule for this year's Outlook day event and the gala evening. I recognised names on the documents of people I had met the year before who were also volunteering. The event was going to be in Oxford, and I pre-booked a pesto and tomato salad, with roast lamb and vegetables for the evening meal.

April 16th 2016

I woke up at 6.30 to have a shower and wash my hair before breakfast. I got my purple TS t-shirt out of my wardrobe, pulled on some skinny jeans and wrapped myself in my long beige cardigan. How much make-up would I put on? There's going to be professional make-up artists coming in for the evening – maybe just my natural brown eyeshadow and my coral lipstick will do?

Before we left, I folded up my dress, found my nude heels and zipped my laptop and camera into their cases for Dad to bring to the hotel this evening.

I felt apprehensive getting into Mum's car. This day was about the very thing I disliked about myself. I can hide my TS away normally, but this day was about celebrating it, and that felt strange. I spoke about my fears to Mum in the car. "I'm normal but I'm not normal. I feel different to people with TS, but I can feel different to people without it too…"

When we arrived at the hotel, Mum dropped me off, wishing me luck and that I have a good time. I returned a small, sad, smile. *I'll try.*

I made my way through the revolving door and found myself in the familiar lobby I had seen when I visited with Dad back in March. There were TSA banners everywhere and the lobby was buzzing full of people; parents, carers and those who had TS as well. Some faces I'd seen before; others that were new. I was worried people may have settled in the night before and that I was going to be left out just coming for the day.

I wandered over to the table where they were handing out lanyards for the event and slid mine on. As I turned around, I received a surprise bear hug from one of the other TS-affected volunteers. I remembered from last year that they were original Outlook members and had been attending the events over the last 20 years. For the first time in the day, I began to relax.

Before the main conference began I was greeted by more familiar faces and spoke to a young woman called Hannah*, and her mum. It was their first time at Outlook this year. Hannah reminded me of myself a few years before, seeming awkward but excited at this strange event with other people who had TS too. I would have never guessed she had the condition from just looking at her.

I found myself explaining to Hannah how welcoming the Outlook community are and that it was my first-time last year. I continued saying that I was now volunteering for the TSA and taking the photos at the gala evening that night. I noticed some copies of Scan on the table opposite and picked one up. "See, this is me on the front," I disclosed bashfully.

Hannah and I discovered that we both attend the same TS clinic and share the same consultant. She also took part in a medical trial I had volunteered for, a few years back, to test if the medicine reduced the size of our TS tumours. It was amazing how animated our conversation was and that I didn't have to explain all the complicated details of the condition that I would have done otherwise. It was refreshing.

The medical research part of the day began at 10:45 after the introductions and greetings. This was my least favourite part of the day. I was transported back to all the squirmy details about brains, lungs and kidneys that I had heard about at the science conference last September, before I remembered that all this research was for people like me; all of us in the room.

I was reminded how everyone with TS is affected differently and which genes can be faulty and whether the TS child will develop Autism, a learning disability or any other impairments.

My curiosity grew when a slide on mental health came up, noting how anxiety can increase around the ages of sixteen-seventeen, which was when my experience of anxiety appeared. *No wonder my anxieties were health-related...*

As I queued up for the indoor barbeque lunch, Tanya, the Volunteer Coordinator, asked me how my job was and said that I looked well. I explained how the Support Worker role really suits me and that I can use my TS experience to help empathise with the people I support – the frustrations they have about up-coming appointments or simply just having a long-term condition. Tanya was really pleased.

After my hot dog I remembered that I had agreed to take part in a video interview that involved many people with TS talking about their experiences of the TSA and Outlook. I followed Tanya to the conference room where the TSA chairman, Rob, had set up a homely corner with set lights and reflectors; photography equipment that I had been used to in my university days. As I sat down on the cosy leather chair, I felt like I was on breakfast tv.

Tanya encouraged me to sit comfortably and I asked her if I needed to look at the camera.
    "Just look at me, that will be fine."
    "I guess that makes sense, seeing as the camera is like the audience's eye." I observed.
    "Exactly," Rob responded, surprised we shared a similar language of technical knowledge.

Tanya explained she didn't need to use any pre-written questions and that the interview would be like an informal conversation. *Perhaps I would have preferred pre-written questions. I'm nervous.*

Rob's video camera began rolling and Tanya asked what it meant for me to be at the 20th Outlook event today. Everything I imagined saying, all those worries and negativity, went out the window. Instead I spoke about the confidence these events were giving me and how being a part of something has helped me feel less alone. As I was talking, I realised that I had been isolating myself by not accepting the advantages of being involved in a support group for such a rare condition. *Why make myself more of an outcast than I need to?*

When Rob and Tanya were happy with the content, I was able to return back to the activities, with a drama therapy workshop about to begin. Although I was part of an amateur dramatics group growing up, Drama reminded me of social awkwardness at secondary school and my niggling doubts about my acting ability. But here, what did I have to feel awkward about? We all had TS and have nothing to hide.

I became more involved with the group activity. Firstly, we talked to the people next to us about our names and then walked around the room smiling at the faces we passed. *This didn't seem too bad.*

After some more group activities, we listened to a speech from one of the founding Outlook members, Corinne. She spoke about what Outlook had meant for her, helping her build confidence, meeting her husband and raising a family despite challenges she had faced. I was intrigued that *outlook* had been chosen for the support group name, because *we look outside to the world from within,* she said. It made me think of looking out of a window, hoping to fit in to the world out there. Corinne continued to say that *outlook* could also be about having a positive outlook on life with TS, and that that strength can increase the more people we share it with.

As Outlook dispersed to get dressed up for the evening, I reflected over Corinne's speech. I hadn't spoken to her much, other than the drama therapy session, but I could instantly relate to how she used to describe herself as being a shy, quiet girl and that that all changed when she came to the Outlook events. She shared how she has learnt to accept herself for who she is and that I have been learning to accept myself too.

1920s Evening

When Dad arrived with my evening clothes, I changed in a toilet cubicle, struggling to gracefully pull up a pair of tights in such a small space. Once dressed I looked at myself in the mirror, topped up my lipstick and smiled; I felt confident in my favourite dress, heels and new hat. I had every reason to feel good. *But was I overdressed?* I swallowed down as much confidence as I could and stepped out of the Ladies into the lobby.

There were a few people from Outlook dotted around, most still in their day clothes, playing pool and having cups of tea.

"Ooh! look at you!?" someone said.
"Don't you look gorgeous."
"Wow!" Came other voices. I smiled bashfully and thanked my admirers and averted my gaze.

I made my way back to the second conference room where the final video interviews were coming to an end. Dad had begun setting up the photography equipment and I gave him a hand. The TSA had ordered a backdrop of a staircase to be used for the photos and after it was put up, Dad took a test picture of me in front of it.

The make-up team arrived for the evening. I asked one of the heavily-made-up women whether I needed to remove the eyeshadow and lipstick I had already applied, but they said they would just go over the top with fresh make-up. In a way I would have preferred starting with a fresh face, but makeovers weren't exactly my thing.

After flicking through some 1920s looks, I pointed to the fourth one; a dramatic forest green eyeshadow with a dark shaded border. "I think that will go great with my dress," I say, imagining I was behind the scenes of a 1920s movie set. It was a great way to continue celebrating my birthday from a few days before.

At first, I enjoyed being pampered. I had mint green eyeshadow base applied over my eyelids, then the darker shades in the corners and along the lash lines. Next came some mascara. This was great. I felt like a princess.

My princess bubble burst when I was asked if I wanted any foundation on my skin. I thought back to being a teenager, trying on that sticky foundation and how it made my complexion worse. I felt self-conscious and hated how close the make-up artist was to my imperfect skin.

"No, thanks," I smile. "Can I have some liquid eyeliner though?"

The lady passed me a mirror after she applied the eyeliner and some berry lipstick. I was surprised by my reflection, feeling more dressed for Halloween, rather than a 1920s dinner. More kind comments seem to fly by, which I could only accept, although I was more confident being behind the camera for the next hour, whilst others had their dressed-up looks done.

It was a relief to find a seat free at a table in the dining area, meeting and speaking to more TS-families I had only acknowledged briefly throughout the day. I talked about my volunteering and my support work for Mencap. I was surprised to hear that the daughter of the family sitting next to me lived in supported living and that she really enjoyed it. It was just so strange that I supported people like Clara* but both of us had TS.

Similarly, I had a conversation with a woman of a similar age to me called Sophie*. She was supporting an Outlook member called Catlin*. Again, I felt the same confusion of my role and who I was; an Outlook attendee like Catlin, but a committed support worker like Sophie, plus a TSA volunteer. Sophie asked me how I became involved with Outlook.

A gasp escaped Sophie's mouth; her eyebrows raised.

"Wow! From the outside, no one would ever think you had TS."

"Thanks," I reply.

Sure, I would expect a comment like that from my family, but from a stranger who doesn't have TS themselves, to genuinely react like that was rather special. But then, with fashion model looks, I wouldn't have imagined Sophie to work in such a caring role. It just showed for both of us that our initial perceptions of each other were quite different.

April 17th 2016

I enjoyed yesterday's Outlook event more than I thought I would. Maybe it's because it's my second year and I felt more a part of the group? Maybe working at Mencap has helped me accept other people with TS too?

The remainder of the year was fairly quiet on the TSA front. There weren't any further events I wanted to take part in, but I was pleased when the photos I had taken from Outlook went on the TSA website. I ordered one Dad took of me in my outfit and placed it in a pearl edged photo frame that now sits on my printer.

TSA 40 Story
November 2016

As the Christmas adverts were beginning to arrive on the tv, I received the winter issue of Scan magazine asking people to send in their stories about their experiences with TS. It was going to be the 40th anniversary of the TSA the next year. I decided to take the plunge and make a start on my next article, focusing less on the volunteering, but what living with TS and LAM is really like for me. The double life I seem to lead; normal until something health-related comes up, but grateful for the medical support I receive.

December

6th December 2016

It was such a relief to finally send off my TSA 40 story. I hope people like it.

Over Christmas, I loved having Geoffrey and Sarah around with their growing families and presents. By Boxing Day, home life was returning back to normal and Mum, Dad and I were recovering from the grandparenting and Auntie duties over the past couple of days. It was good to have some relaxation time in my room, reading my new books and putting away my presents. Mum came upstairs and told me she had a surprise for me that she'd forgotten to give out the day before.

I followed her downstairs and opened the cotton drawstring bag in front of me. I reached in and picked up a squishy 30cm tall crocheted doll. *That's me! That's me in my 1920s outfit – the brown cloche hat, my hair, the dress, the shoes...*

"Alison made it for you," explained Mum, describing how our neighbour was inspired to make the doll once she saw my photo.

As I held the doll in my hands, admiring the dark beads for my eyes and all the details, the realisation hit that, if I didn't have TS or hadn't attended this year's Outlook event, I probably wouldn't be owning a personalised doll made for me, of me.

2017

At the start of the year I celebrated my second working year with Mencap and began taking the new medication that would reduce the size of my TS and LAM tumours. This year's Outlook event would be in September, so my interest in photography and volunteering was dwindling.

September

At the start of the month I began my second counselling course and attended Outlook on the 23rd. I had felt lost in myself over the year. I still felt apprehensive about the TS community but grateful that such a community did exist. School friends were leaving home and getting married. Other than my counselling career, I didn't know what I was supposed to be doing at twenty-four.

Whereas I wrote in great detail about the two previous Outlook events, the journal page of that day remained blank. I attended the event, but I didn't volunteer. I took part in the creative art class that celebrated 40 years of the TSA; a vibrant square image of a smile. But was I smiling on the inside?

As much as these activities were designed for the group to connect with each other, I couldn't help but feel patronised. *Can't we just talk to each other like adults? Talk about our TS experiences or just what we've been up to? Do we have to do child-like drawings? This is not what I come to these events for.*

A few weeks later the autumnal issue of Scan flopped through my letterbox. I recognised the glittery, smiley canvas I had made at Outlook, which was now part of a collage magazine cover of other bright artworks from the day. I returned a small appreciative grin towards it.

As always, I flicked through the magazine and spotted extracts from the TSA 40 stories, mine at the bottom of the double-paged-spread. I read my words *double life* and typed in the link to the stories onto the website.

I revisited my article I had sent to off to the TSA at the end of 2016. More words and phrases highlighting themselves to me:

"To the outside world, no one would suspect I have TS..."

"When I go to my appointments, I'm reminded I have TS and LAM...it feels horrible to recognise that I might not always be normal."

"I've been trying to understand for a long time whether I'm normal or not, but it's just best to go with being me. I am fluid person, a mixture of normality, TS and LAM."

"I have gained confidence in myself that I never knew I had..."

Outlook, the TSA and Career Article
2018

My confidence seemed to fluctuate. I was getting closer to accepting myself but from time to time still wanted to resist TS and LAM. The Outlook event this year was up north, and I didn't feel like travelling all that way. At the same time it was a relief. I didn't have to commit to every Outlook event if I didn't want to and thought maybe a break from it would do me some good.

When I began the first year of my Level 4 counselling diploma, it was through my personal counselling sessions that I began to realise the resistance I had against my health conditions and that other affected people were reminders of what I've got. They were me, but not me, like distorted reflections in a hall of mirrors. In my mind I would be running away from them, but like on a treadmill, not moving anywhere.

2019

Bristol seemed a lot easier to get to by train than Manchester, so I chose to go to the 2019 Outlook event. Having stepped back last year, reflecting over my resistance through therapy, I felt more tolerant of TS and the Outlook group around me.

19th May 2019

I met some old and new faces and felt more confident again. I remembered I didn't have to hide my TS, and I enjoyed cutting and sticking magazine scraps to create collages of ourselves - "See me, not TSC".

July

In the summer I received an unexpected email from the TSA about a new section of their website that they will be hosting from September. They wanted as many real-life accounts of people living with TS as possible, but as I had already done that, I decided to write about how TS and LAM have influenced my career.

I wrote about the connections of wanting to be a nurse growing up, influenced by my hospital appointments; Helen with Cerebral Palsy, and working for Mencap; the CBT I had for Health Anxiety that led me to become a counsellor, and of course volunteering for the TSA. It was great to see another article on their website. I was finally integrating my conditions positively and using my experiences to empathise with others through my professions.

2020

I knew the Outlook event had to move around the country every couple of years so that mildly affected adults with TS could access it when it came to them. This year it was going to be in Durham, and like 2018, I didn't have the emotional energy to travel that far. There was always social media if I wanted to chat to any of the Outlook members before another event came around that was more local.

Rare Disease Day & Acceptance

February

Rare Disease Day takes always takes place on the last day of February. I feel grateful that it is acknowledged as an awareness day, but honestly, I probably wouldn't know it existed if I wasn't affected by two rare diseases myself. In a way, it's rare for people to know about TS or LAM if they haven't been influenced by either condition personally or know of someone who is affected.

29th February 2020

I can't deny how guilty I feel. It's Rare Disease Day and I'm realising more and more why I've struggled to connect to the Outlook group. Some members posted a quote on Facebook about "see the person first, not the condition." I connected to that quote so much because I don't want TS to define me and I do want to be seen as a person first. But in some horrible ironic way, I had labelled Outlook as a group of people who just had TS, not showing the curiosity to get to know them as individuals.

Alone in my room, I felt shameful for my subconscious judgements. I realised that I had been judging the group for an aspect that I judged in myself; and that's when it all made sense. Genuinely I did want to connect to Outlook, but by disassociating myself from them I only increased my isolation rather than connection. Like my appointment days, Outlook was one of those occasions where I had to look TS in the face and admit to myself, once again, I have it. But if I was beginning to accept myself, then perhaps it would be easier to accept the group as warm-hearted people, who just happen to have TS too. In connection I noticed I had similar unconscious, unfair judgements about LAM-affected people too.

March

In order to develop better social connections with both TS and LAM, I made some notes about how I could go about that.

Notes
- *Remain curious.*
- *What is beyond each person at Outlook other than TS?*
- *What makes them who they are?*
- *What are their interests?*
- *What are their values?*

What is beyond each person with LAM?
- *What makes them who they are?*
- *What are their interests?*
- *What are their values?*

I thought about the curiosity that my counselling placement supervisor was encouraging. That by being curious, we show an interest in a person's life and that makes them feel valued. Everyone wants to feel valued. I thought about my clients at my placement and despite all the various backgrounds; the various upbringings; the difference and diversity, I had little judgement for them. I had little judgement for the people I supported at Mencap. They didn't have TS and LAM, so I could connect to them and understand them. By deciding to put the conditions to one side, it was like releasing a padlock to a heavy metal barrier I had placed between myself and other TS/LAM affected people. I was now in a place where I could gradually start expressing that curiosity and develop empathy and understanding for those who have had similar life-experiences to me. It was freeing.

April

In the midst of the first Coronavirus Lockdown, with many having to shield from the outside world, Outlook 2020, was rearranged to an online video call. For the first time in a long time, I felt like I wanted to attend.

Although I contributed sometimes, for the most part I was an observer. I watched the gallery of over thirty faces looking back at me. There was nothing wrong with them really. I just hadn't given them a chance. *We all have TS and I could see many intelligent and able people chatting away.*

Throughout the lockdown period some of the regular Outlook members suggested a regular video call pub-quiz; and again, I felt more inclined to join in. I saw these online meetings were opportunities to exercise my curiosity in an informal setting and get to know these people who have TS, without having to focus the discussion on the condition itself.

At times I held back and chose which weeks I wanted to join in or have space to recharge. But when I did, I was being that observer again; cautious about how to be in the group. I could see how supportive everyone was of each other, while casually mocking difficult general knowledge questions. There was friendship there.

I noticed that despite not knowing some of the answers to the questions myself, I was impressed with how much knowledge everyone came with and how I had previously underestimated the overall intelligence of the group.

I was made to feel welcomed and that was really touching. Nonetheless, I wondered whether I really did deserve that kindness after my previously hidden judgements. Although it may have seemed that I was judging them, I knew deep down it was about how I was judging myself. And I didn't want to judge myself anymore and I didn't want to judge anyone with TS or LAM either.

April, 2021

Our beautiful, brave daughter, Zoë, died on Easter Monday. Not as a result of her anxiety which she had overcome, nor of her Tuberous Sclerosis or LAM which she confronted daily, but from lymphoma which had developed rapidly. She put up a courageous fight against it and was actually looking forward to the chemo because she could see a better life for herself in the future. However, out of the blue, she had a cardiac arrest resulting in massive brain damage which led to her death five days later.

In true Zoë form, she was WhatsApping her friends and family in high spirits just hours before the cardiac arrest, leaving us all with a happy image of the amazing girl that we will cherish for ever.

We would like to thank not only the doctors, nurses and staff on this occasion in the ICU, the Adelaide ward and the Cardiac Care Unit, at the Royal Berkshire Hospital, Reading, for their skills, knowledge and unstinting care, but also those at her Bath, Nottingham and Oxford clinics, and her GP, Doctor Keast. They always gave Zoë, the very best of themselves and are a shining example of the NHS.

---

*Denotes name changed to protect identity

References

Opening Quote

Company, W.D (1998) *Walt Disney Company Quotes* Accessed 2020: https://www.goodreads.com/author/quotes/3510823.Walt_Disney_Company

Introduction

Lexico. s.d *Anomoly*. Accessed 2020: https://www.lexico.com/definition/anomaly

Sunderland, A.T (1981) *Disabled We Stand. Chapter 6: Stereotypes of Disability*. Accessed 2020: https://disability-studies.leeds.ac.uk/wp-content/uploads/sites/40/library/Sutherland-CHAPTER6.pdf

Tuberous Sclerosis Association (2019) *What is TSC?* Accessed 2020: https://tuberous-sclerosis.org/information-and-support/what-is-tsc/

"Sclerosis." *Merriam-Webster.com Dictionary*, Merriam-Webster, https://www.merriam-webster.com/dictionary/sclerosis.Accessed 2020.

MS Society.s.d. *What is MS?* Accessed 2020: https://www.mssociety.org.uk/about-ms/what-is-ms?gclid=CjwKCAiA4o79BRBvEiwAjteoYD_4g_oLW-WZHx5UZ0OMJ-EbOPZp0rigz2UA7Wrt-0a7Gh2JH5i7VBoCoGcQAvD_BwE

Tuberous Sclerosis Association (2019) *TSC and Genetics.* Accessed 2020: https://tuberous-sclerosis.org/information-and-support/tsc-and-genetics/

N. s.d. *What is DNA?* Accessed 2020: https://www.your genome.org/facts/what-is-dna

Medline Plus. (2018) *Tuberous Sclerosis Complex.* Accessed 2020: https://medlineplus.gov/genetics/condition/tuberous-sclerosis-complex/#sourcesforpage

Medline Plus. (2018) *TSC 1 Gene.* Accessed 2020: https://medlineplus.gov/genetics/gene/tsc1/#conditions

McGlynne, F. (2019) *Genetics and TSC.* Accessed 2020: https://tuberous-sclerosis.org/wp-content/uploads/2019/10/TSA-TSC-and-genetics.pdf

McGlynee, F (2019) *An Introduction to Tuberous Sclerosis Complex.* Accessed 2020: https://tuberous-sclerosis.org/wp-content/uploads/2019/10/TSA-An-introduction-to-TSC.pdf

Medline Plus. (2018) *Lymphangioleimyomatosis.* Accessed 2020: https://medlineplus.gov/genetics/condition/lymphangiol eiomyomatosis/#diagnosis

Chapter 1

World Health Organisation. (2019) *Epilepsy.* Accessed 2020: https://www.who.int/news-room/fact-sheets/detail/epilepsy

Epilepsy Action. s.d. *Absence Seizures.* Accessed 2020: https://www.epilepsy.org.uk/info/seizures/absence-seizures

Epilepsy Action. s.d. *What is Epilepsy?* Accessed 2020: https://www.epilepsy.org.uk/info/what-is-epilepsy

Epilepsy Society (2018) *Focal Impaired Awareness Seizures.* Accessed 2020: https://epilepsysociety.org.uk/focal-impaired-awareness-seizures#.XnuFMi2cbOQ

Tuberous Sclerosis Association (2019) *Epilepsy*. Accessed 2020: https://tuberous-sclerosis.org/tsc_affects_the_body/epilepsy/

Tuberous Sclerosis Association (2019) *Brain*. Accessed 2020: https://tuberous-sclerosis.org/tsc_affects_the_body/brain/

NHS. (2018) *MRI Scan*. Accessed 2020: https://www.nhs.uk/conditions/mri-scan/

Chapter 2

Tuberous Sclerosis Association (2019) *Skin*. Accessed 2020: https://tuberous-sclerosis.org/tsc_affects_the_body/skin/

NHS (2018) *Treatment: Tuberous Sclerosis*. Accessed 2020: https://www.nhs.uk/conditions/tuberous-sclerosis/treatment/

Health Line (2018) *Laser Therapy: Purpose, Procedure and Risks*. Accessed 2020: https://www.healthline.com/health/laser-therapy

Teng, J. (2013) *Skin*. Accessed 2020: https://www.tsalliance.org/about-tsc/signs-and-symptoms-of-tsc/skin/

Chapter 3

NIH (2018) *Your Kidneys and How they Work*. Accessed 2020: https://www.niddk.nih.gov/health-information/kidney-disease/kidneys-how-they-work

Tuberous Sclerosis Association (2019) *Kidneys*. Accessed 2020: https://tuberous-sclerosis.org/tsc_affects_the_body/kidneys/

The LAM Foundation. sd. *What is LAM?* Accessed 2020: https://www.thelamfoundation.org/Newly-Diagnosed/Learning-About-Lam/About-LAM

NHS (2019) *Blood Transfusion*. Accessed 2020: https://www.nhs.uk/conditions/blood-transfusion/

Chapter 4

LAM Action. s.d. *What are the Symptoms of LAM*. Accessed 2020: http://lamaction.org/about-lam/what-are-the-symptoms-of-lam/

Johnson, S and Tattersfield, A. (2019) *Lymphangioleimyomatosis: LAM Fact Sheet*. Accessed 2020: http://lamaction.org/wp-content/uploads/2019/02/LAM-Fact-Sheet-2019.pdf

Tuberous Sclerosis Association (2019) *Lungs*. Accessed 2020: https://tuberous-sclerosis.org/tsc_affects_the_body/lungs/

Nottingham University Hospital NHS Trust. s.d. *National Centre for LAM*. Accessed 2020. https://www.nuh.nhs.uk/national-centre-for-lam

Healthline (2017) *Pulmonary Function Test*. Accessed 2020. https://www.nuh.nhs.uk/national-centre-for-lam

NHS (2018) *CT Scan*. Accessed 2020. https://www.nhs.uk/conditions/ct-scan/

LAM Action. s.d. *National Centre for LAM*. Accessed 2020: http://lamaction.org/for-patients-their-families/uk-national-centre-for-lam/

University of Nottingham. s.d. *School of Medicine: Simon Johnson*. Accessed 2020: https://www.nottingham.ac.uk/medicine/people/simon.johnson

Ballou, L.M and Lin, R.Z. (2008) *Rapamycin and mTOR Kinase Inhibitors*. Accessed 2020. https://www.ncbi.nlm.nih.gov/pmc/articles/PMC2698317/

LAM Action. s.d. *Our Story*. Accessed 2020: http://lamaction.org/about-lam-action/our-story/

Chapter 5

Tuberous Sclerosis Association (2019) *TSC-Associated Neuropsychiatric Disorders (TAND)*. Accessed 2020: https://

tuberous-sclerosis.org/tsc_affects_the_body/tsc-associated-neuropsychiatric-disorders-tand/

NHS (2018) *Attention Deficient Hyperactivity Disorder (ADHD).* Accessed 2020. https://www.nhs.uk/conditions/attention-deficit-hyperactivity-disorder-adhd/

NHS (2018) *General Anxiety Disorder in Adults.* Accessed 2020. https://www.nhs.uk/conditions/generalised-anxiety-disorder/

Head, E. (2018) *What is the difference between Stress and Anxiety?* Accessed 2020. https://www.nhs.uk/conditions/generalised-anxiety-disorder/

Mind. s.d. *What is stress?* Accessed 2020. https://www.mind.org.uk/information-support/types-of-mental-health-problems/stress/what-is-stress/

Mind. s.d. *What is anxiety?* Accessed 2020. https://www.mind.org.uk/information-support/types-of-mental-health-problems/anxiety-and-panic-attacks/about-anxiety/#WhatIsTheFightFlightOrFreezeResponse

Mind. s.d. *Anxiety and Panic Attacks. Accessed 2020. https://www.mind.org.uk/information-support/types-of-mental-health-problems/anxiety-and-panic-attacks/anxiety-symptoms*

McLeod, S. (2019) Cognitive Behavioural Therapy. Accessed 2020. https://www.simplypsychology.org/cognitive-therapy.html

NHS (2019) *Cognitive Behavioural Therapy.* Accessed 2020. https://www.nhs.uk/conditions/cognitive-behavioural-therapy-cbt/

Brainy Quote. s.d *Epictetus Quotes.* Accessed 2020. https://www.brainyquote.com/quotes/epictetus_149126

Chapter 6

Tuberous Sclerosis Association (2019) *Education*. Accessed 2020. https://tuberous-sclerosis.org/life-with-tsc/education/

Tuberous Sclerosis Association (2019) *Early Years and Childhood*. Accessed 2020. https://tuberous-sclerosis.org/life-with-tsc/early-years-and-childhood/

Kumon. s.d. *About Kumon*. Accessed 2020. https://www.kumon.co.uk/about/

Chapter 7

Mencap. s.d. *Mencap's History*. Accessed 2020. https://www.mencap.org.uk/about-us/mencaps-history

Mencap. s.d. *Supported Living Services*. Accessed 2020. https://www.mencap.org.uk/advice-and-support/services-you-can-count/supported-living-services

LDA. s.d. *Types of Learning Disabilities*. Accessed 2020. https://ldaamerica.org/types-of-learning-disabilities/

Lowth, M and Bonsall, A. (2016) *General Learning Disability. Accessed 2020. https://patient.info/doctor/general-learning-disability*

Tuberous Sclerosis Association (2019) *Intellectual Ability*. Accessed 2020. https://tuberous-sclerosis.org/tsc_affects_the_body/intellectual-ability/

Kare Plus (2017) *Care and Support; What is the difference?* Accessed 2020. https://kareplus.co.uk/wolverhampton/2017/08/21/care-support-whats-the-difference/

National Careers Service. s.d. *National Careers Service*. Accessed 2020. https://nationalcareers.service.gov.uk

Chapter 8

BACP .s.d *Careers in Counselling*. Accessed 2020: https://www.bacp.co.uk/careers/careers-in-counselling/

Mind (2020) https://www.mind.org.uk

Biography (2017) *Sigmund Freud*. Accessed 2020. *https://www.biography.com/scholar/sigmund-freud*

Tavistock and Portman NHS Trust. sd. *History. Accessed 2020. https://tavistockandportman.nhs.uk/about-us/who-we-are/history/*

Tavistock and Portman NHS Trust .s.d. *Introduction to Counselling and Psychotherapy.* Accessed 2020. https://tavistockandportman.nhs.uk/training/courses/introduction-counselling-and-psychotherapy-d12/

Davies, J. (2015) *Pyschological Splitting and How You May Be Using It Without Even Knowing.* Accessed 2020. https://www.learning-mind.com/psychological-splitting/

Queensborough Community College. s.d. *Definition for Diversity.* Accessed 2020. https://www.qcc.cuny.edu/diversity/definition.html

Counselling and Psychotherapy Training Academy (2020) https://www.cpta.org.uk

Books
- Person-Centred Counselling in Action. 4th edition – Mearns, Thorne and McLeod.
- First Steps in Counselling. 4th edition – Pete Sanders.
- Integrative Counselling in Action. 3rd ed. – Culley and Bond
- A Short Introduction to Psychoanalysis. 2nd ed. – Jane Milton
- Client Centred Therapy – Carl R. Rogers

- Draw On Your Emotions. 2nd ed. – Margot Sunderland
- Braving the Wilderness – Brené Brown

Chapter 9

Tuberous Sclerosis Association (2019) *History of the TSA.* Accessed 2020. https://tuberous-sclerosis.org/about-the-tsa/ history-of-the-tsa/

Tuberous Sclerosis Association (2020) *Outlook.* Accessed 2020. https://tuberous-sclerosis.org/get-involved/our-community-events/outlook-virtual-meeting-2020/

Tuberous Sclerosis Association (2019) *Family Fun Days.* Accessed 2020. https://tuberous-sclerosis.org/get-involved/ our-community-events/family-fun-days/

Tuberous Sclerosis Assoication (2019) *Community Groups.* Accessed 2020. https://tuberous-sclerosis.org/get-involved/ community-groups-and-other-groups/